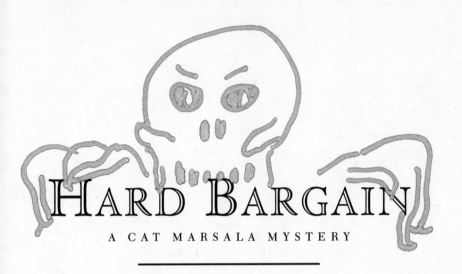

HARD BARGAIN

A CAT MARSALA MYSTERY

Barbara D'Amato

To Joanie
The Finest!

Barbara D'Amato

SCRIBNER

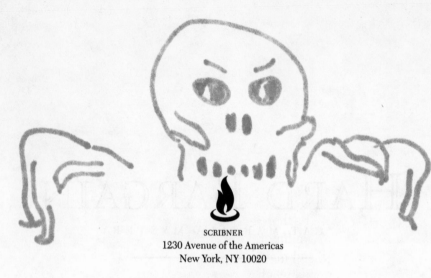

SCRIBNER
1230 Avenue of the Americas
New York, NY 10020

A joint venture with
Berkley Publishing Group
200 Madison Avenue
New York, NY 10020

Set in Caledonia

Manufactured in the United States of America

1 3 5 7 9 10 8 6 4 2

Library of Congress Cataloging-in-Publication Data
D'Amato, Barbara.
Hard bargain : a Cat Marsala mystery / Barbara D'Amato.
p.   cm.
1. Marsala, Cat (Fictitious character)—Fiction. I. Title.
PS3554.A4674H32   1997
813'.54—dc21   97-20622
CIP

ISBN 0-684-83353-0

Through the years there has been one person who has helped in every way—finding reference material, advising on legal, mathematical, and many other matters, and especially reading drafts and giving advice and creative suggestions. I want to thank Tony D'Amato.

HARD BARGAIN

◆ 1 ◆

I dropped my coat on the chair and pushed the door behind me closed with the heel of my left foot. It was 9 A.M. on an oppressively beautiful, warm Tuesday morning in March. A nice long nap was in order. What a night! I was riding with the midnight-to-8-A.M. shift, working on a story about emergency medical technicians, EMTs.

Long John Silver, my parrot, swooped in from the bedroom and tried to land on my hair. He thinks pulling hair is amusing. I waved him away. He settled onto the sofa arm instead and said, "But look, the morn, in russet mantle clad, walks o'er the dew of yon high eastern hill."

I said, "You idiot, that's the Sears Tower."

He said, "Braaaak!"

"I'd better check the messages before I collapse," I told him. Somebody might be offering me an assignment to interview Queen Elizabeth, all expenses paid. Or maybe a survey of the three-plus star restaurants of Aspen, Colorado. It was equally likely I'd exhale fast and rocket to Jupiter. All that editors wanted from me was crime and conflagration.

Five messages on the machine.

Beep. "Uh, hi, Cat. Um—this is Teddy—how are you? I was just calling—um—to ask whether you could do me a favor."

My brother. *Love you a lot, but get on with it. I need sleep.*

"Could you send me a copy of that book on the Los Angeles Police Department? It sounds great. When you get a chance, give me a call. Call soon because Mom is all cranked up wanting us to come to dinner next Sunday. Bye."

I sank into the sofa. *Beep.* Next message.

"Cat? Are you there?" Pause. "Well, okay, I'm delighted you're out working for me. This is your friendly editor, Hal Briskman. Can you speed up that article? Turns out Henrietta fell through and we need your piece three days early. She fell through literally, by the way. Overfilled her waterbed and it went straight down into the apartment below. Swamped a burglar, actually, and the bed held him in place until the police and ambulance came. That's our Henrietta. But her laptop fell in with her and shorted out. Lost all her files. So get me that article chop-chop." Hal loves antique slang. When he's pleased with me he tells me I'm the bee's knees.

He hung up without saying good-bye. He's only good at punctuation on paper. I gnashed my teeth briefly, but I'm trying to train myself out of this habit and hastily slapped myself on the cheek instead.

Beep.

"Cat, this is John. I'm at La Guardia. Ought to hit O'Hare by midday. Hong Kong was nice, but Da Vinci was a nightmare. I'm glad to be back. We've been separated too long. We need to get together and talk. I'll call tonight."

My significant other. Deal with that later.

"Ms. Marsala, this is Mr. Whillis."

My landlord. Great! Maybe he was finally going to fix the leak over the bedroom window. I leaned farther back into the sofa.

"Your existing lease will be up in two months. If you wish to renew, tell me within fifteen days. And by the way, I will be raising rents in the building thirty percent."

AAARGHHH! I sank farther into the sofa and started to gnash my teeth again.

Beep.

"Cat, this is Bramble in Chief McCoo's office. He needs help and he's too proud to ask. Would you come to the office as soon as you can?"

I sat bolt upright. My friend Harold McCoo is the Chicago

Police Department's chief of detectives. In ten years of friend-ship, he has *never* asked for my help. He's never needed my help. And he has helped me with cases a hundred times.

Rubbing exhaustion out of my eyes, I jumped up and ran for the door.

The Central Administration of the Chicago Police Depart-ment is located at Eleventh and State, a mile south of the Loop in an area of patchy dilapidation and regentrification. The building was built in the 1920s and looks it.

McCoo's office is on the eighth floor in the main building, down a corridor of speckled brown linoleum, the kind designed not to show dirt by the crafty trick of looking very much as if it's already dirty.

There are double doors leading into an anteroom, then another set of doors leading into the main office of the chief of detectives. The arrangement wastes valuable space, but that's an old building for you. The main office is maybe twenty by thirty feet. McCoo's secretary, Bramble, sits at a large wooden desk against the wall on your left as you come in. Against the wall on the right, the outside wall with the win-dows in it, are three somewhat smaller desks. The one nearest the front door is Russell Lupinski's. The middle one is Tracy Shoemaker's. And the back one, near the file cabinets, is Fred Koy's. So you face the whole support staff the instant you walk in the door. The windows are industrial glass reinforced with chicken wire. They were last washed to celebrate the end of the blackout after World War Two.

The entry door to McCoo's private office is toward the back, directly behind Bramble and across from Koy.

Despite the unedifying surroundings and the dim quality of the outdoor light that these windows let in, this little band is usually quite jolly. McCoo is an understanding boss. He requires hard work and a high level of accuracy, but rewards with approval. And he picks staff who are naturally precise people.

"Hi, guys," I said.

They stared glumly at me. Finally, Bramble said, "Thanks for coming."

Where was the cheerful backchat? The good-natured joshing?

"Well, sure," I said. "So how are you all doing?"

Koy said, "Not great."

"Mmm, is Chief McCoo busy?"

They stared glumly at me. Then Bramble said, "No. He isn't. Not exactly."

"Should I just go in?"

"Could you, please?" she said drearily.

I looked at her, then at Koy, Lupinski, and Shoemaker, but none of them explained, and finally I just walked past them into McCoo's office.

McCoo stood at his window. His coffeemaker was cold. There was no smell of Ethiopian harrar or Kenyan brune or Sumatra mandheling. Cautiously, I said, "Hi."

"Oh, Cat. What are you doing here?"

The voice lacked expression. McCoo is African-American, tall but slightly overweight, rather scholarly-looking. Today his face was stony. The set of his shoulders was stiff.

"Bramble called me."

"Mmmmp." It sounded as if he thought Bramble was taking too much into her own hands.

A coffee mug stood on his desk. I said, "Want me to make some coffee?" I was exhausted from my long night, and some caffeine-booster wouldn't hurt, especially one of McCoo's excellent coffees. And McCoo obviously needed a cup.

"They've got some instant outside," he said. Aghast, I turned back to the door. "Bring some coffee creamer, too," he said.

I stepped back into the main office, half-aware that I was tiptoeing. "He wants—uh—instant coffee and coffee creamer?" I said, as a question, not a statement.

The four in the office stared at me with wide eyes. They knew even better than I that McCoo was the world's greatest coffee gourmet. In his office he had a Scandinavian pot, a Krups grinder, and a tiny refrigerator that stocked real, fresh cream. Tracy Shoemaker got up without a word and handed me a jar of non-dairy creamer. Bramble, rolling her eyes, handed me a jar of instant coffee.

For some reason, we were in deep trouble.

"Okay," I said, "what's the matter?" I stirred powdered coffee whitener—not a tasty description for food—into a cup of instant and handed it to him. I made another for myself and sipped it. It was truly evil. Funny how the mind works. This coffee, which I would cheerfully have consumed when on a rush assignment in the *Chicago Today* offices, tasted hideous when drunk three feet from a bag of glossy Bolivian beans and the shining lure of a Krups grinder.

McCoo grimaced but drank a swallow of his. I repeated, "What's going on?"

Genuinely puzzled, he said, "Have you been living under a rock for the last ten days, Cat?" He pushed a stack of newspapers across his desk to me, studying my face.

"As a matter of fact, for the last week and a half I've slept all day and been up all night with paramedics in their spiffy high-tech emergency vehicles. I get home, feed Long John Silver, plug my notes from my tapes or notepads into my word processor for an hour or so, and go to bed."

"But you must read the papers."

People who are not reporters think that reporters spend all their time reading papers, like stockbrokers watch each other's buys and sells. "I don't have to keep up on every word my colleagues of the Fourth Estate commit to print," I said grandly. "Actually, I scanned the news, and I saw something about a police shooting, if that's what you mean. But, McCoo, I've been really rushed and really pretty tired—"

He sighed. Since he apparently was not coping very well, I pulled the papers closer to me and started reading.

They built in size and violence, like Bruce Lee's opponents in *Game of Death*. The first article was just a quarter column at the bottom of an inside page, dated Monday, March 10, just over a week ago. After a minute, I said, "Oh, hell!"

The gist of the rather short article was that a female police officer had shot a male police officer at his home in the presence of his four-year-old daughter. It suggested that the department was trying to cover up this fact and that the details were being buried "deep in the office of the chief of detectives."

The second sheet was dated a day later, carried a larger headline about the case, set higher on the page. A third paper dated a day after that sported an even larger headline, DIS-CREPANCIES HINTED IN POLICE SHOOTING, and was the lead story, though in a less-important paper.

I threw the first sheets down and picked up two more. The corner of the first clipped McCoo's cup and sent it rolling. Coffee with half-dissolved whitener splattered, making bird droppings across the desk.

"Wasn't worth drinking anyhow," McCoo said, dumping some paper napkins on the splatters.

The *Chicago Times'* Monday, March 17, headline read, SHOOTING PROBE WIDENS. I scanned the text and found:

> The Chicago Police Department investigation of Officer Shelly Daniello, adjourned pending further investigation, will be broadened to include testimony from the department ballistics expert and a physician from the Office of the Cook County Medical Examiner as well as the radio dispatcher and possibly other officers called to the scene after the shooting occurred.
>
> "Yes, this hearing will go beyond the usual round-table inquiry, which we always hold after an officer fires a gun," said Nolly Johnson, acting director of News Affairs for the

Chicago Police Department. Johnson declined further comment, saying that he would not "prejudge a matter under review."

Confidential sources confirm that discrepancies have been noted between Officer Daniello's account of the events surrounding the shooting of her brother-in-law and the physical evidence. Officer Daniello reportedly claims to have fired at Officer Jurack from a distance of three or four feet. But tests of Jurack's clothing confirm that powder burns or residue patterns strongly suggest a distance of "from one foot to point-blank range."

Officer Daniello was placed on suspension after shooting and killing Officer Ben Jurack. Jurack, a fifteen-year veteran of the department, was in a room off his kitchen when he was shot. Jurack was married to Officer Daniello's sister, Marie D. Jurack. Sources say that Officer Daniello was on patrol with her partner, Bradford Hubner, when they received a domestic-violence call to the home of her sister and brother-in-law. The *Times* has learned from the neighbor who placed the initial 911 call that the Juracks had previous domestic-violence incidents—

"Don't worry about the *Chicago Slimes*, McCoo," I said. "Real reporters use it to line birdcages."

"Keep reading," was all he said.

Allegations of spousal abuse by police officers have surfaced frequently over the years, including several high-profile cases recently. The department has always denied any widespread problem. "These are isolated incidents," said Superintendent Ralph Spurlark, "no different from what you would find in any population of twelve thousand individuals."

But reliable sources say that domestic violence has long been a problem in police departments, Chicago not excepted. The *Times* has learned that a special program has been instituted for trainees, intended to warn them of the dangers of anger at home produced by stresses on the job, and presumably giving them techniques for dealing with anger and the desire to do violence.

"It isn't enough," said Jeanette Eady, chair of the Battered Women's Coalition. "We need more active response by the police to scenes of domestic violence in which an officer is involved. Typically, a couple of his fellow officers arrive, take the wife-beater aside, counsel him to 'cool down,' and leave. If the wife insists on their following up, they tell her to think it over awhile first."

Next I picked up a *Tribune* from a few days earlier, Thursday, March 13.

The head read: CHIEF OF DETECTIVES COVERING SLOPPY INVESTIGATION?

The subhead was worse: OR IS THE EXPLANATION MORE SINISTER?

Reliable sources have revealed that Police Officer Ben Jurack, shot last week by a fellow officer, may have been struck on the head before he was shot.

A highly informed source told the *Tribune* that a bruise on the head of Officer Jurack was made "perimortally" or close to the time of death and consisted of "a well-defined purple area associated with a slight swelling .5–1.0 cm wide and 3 cm long . . . 3 cm above the orbital margin." The source would not speculate whether Jurack had in fact been stunned and then shot.

Hanford Reston, long a critic of the police department, said today, "Errors are made in reporting, just like errors are made in investigations. But oftentimes what seems like sloppy reporting may be a premeditated effort to keep the public from learning embarrassing facts."

"Wait a minute," I said. "Let me get all this straight. Officer Shelly Daniello was on regular, normal patrol in a squad car, right?"

"Right."

"She and her partner were given a domestic violence call, to an address which she had to know was her sister's house. Is she supposed to respond to that call or should she have asked another car to go on it?"

"If she's the car that gets the call, she's supposed to go. And act professionally."

"Okay. She finds this Jurack beating her sister, and she shoots him."

"Right. Stabbing her sister, actually."

"Well, I can see why there would be questions. Like, did she *have* to shoot him?"

"That's the biggest question of all. I think she probably did. I think it was a good shooting."

"Did she warn him first?"

"Yes."

"Was he actually threatening the sister with death and had he already done bodily harm?"

"Yes. Bodily harm for sure."

"Where was her partner while she was shooting her brother-in-law?"

"He says he got to the room after Daniello had fired at Jurack. Why he took so long is one of a whole lot of unanswered questions."

"And of course, your people are investigating. The Detective Division investigates cases for the department and Internal Affairs and so on, right?"

"Right."

"And since you're in charge, whatever ax anybody has to grind, they can make you the bad guy. They can claim you're being too hard on Shelly Daniello because she shot a police officer. Or too easy on her because she's a police officer. Or too hard on her because male officers stick together. And so on."

"Right."

"Or that the evidence wasn't properly collected in the first place."

"Or even, God forbid, that somebody planted evidence. Fortunately, nobody's said that yet."

"Or you're covering up as much dirt as possible so the department won't look bad."

"That, certainly. And in fact I have to keep some data confidential. We need to have it uncontaminated for the board inquiry."

"Yeah, I can see this is a can of worms. Whatever you do, you'll be criticized."

"Have *been* criticized."

"Can't you fight back in the press?"

"Not without knowing the facts. I don't actually know what happened at Jurack's. All I know now is that we collected the evidence properly."

"McCoo, you've been criticized before. It's part of the job."

"Investigations get criticized, especially heater cases. But personally, no. I haven't ever really been attacked like this."

"So you've been lucky. Or actually, you've probably been treated the way you deserve. You do your job well, McCoo. And I think the press realizes that and knows you play fair with them. So I suppose you ought to take this as just a small wave in otherwise calm seas."

"That's not the problem."

"Well, what is, then? I hate to see you so depressed, but frankly, I don't think of you as the sort of person who wilts at the first blast of criticism."

"And I hope I'm not. The problem is this. You noticed those 'confidential sources' and 'reliable sources' and so on?"

"Sure."

"The leaks are coming from inside the department."

Pause.

"Hmm," I said. "So who wants your job?"

◇ 3 ◇

"I'm not sure it's my job," he said.

I looked blankly at him, saying "explain" with my eyes. He didn't respond.

"Why would the department want to discredit you? If you look bad, they look bad."

"I didn't say it *was* the department. I said it was somebody *inside* the department. You're absolutely right that accusations like this make the CPD look bad. But somebody doesn't care. Somebody wants to shoot me down in flames—personally."

"Why?"

"Cat, this is Chicago."

"Oh. Politics."

"Politics. The mayor is shaky and the election is coming up in a matter of days. Part of the mayor's problem is that nobody likes the job Spurlark is doing."

Ralph Spurlark was the Superintendent of Police, and to say that nobody liked the job he was doing was like saying people take a dim view of botulism. Spurlark had been able, amazingly enough, to alienate both the get-tough-on-crime people and the civil liberties camp. Not in the same breath, of course. He'd recently visited Russia on a U.S. top-cops tour. When he got home he offered this opinion on "News Nine": "United States law enforcement could learn something from the Russians. Those people have the right idea about how to deal with criminals."

The screams from the liberals over that remark had

scarcely begun to fade when the right end of the political spectrum was dismayed to hear Spurlark say: "We should get a list of all the NRA gun nuts and get warrants and pay them a little home visit and yank their weapons."

McCoo said, "The mayor could replace Spurlark at any moment, and hope that will give him more votes. He's probably trying to decide whether it will help or whether it will look like he should never have appointed Spurlark in the first place. If he decides that, he'll wait until he's reelected. If he's reelected, he'll still probably have to replace Spurlark. Now that we don't have primaries, the election is gonna be a free-for-all. Chester Malling would have a real chance to upset the mayor, if it weren't for Halliby splitting the vote."

All three were Democrats. In Chicago, the Republican mayoral contender usually gets vote percentages in the single digits. Ignoring the Republican, polls showed the race was between the mayor and Malling. We now have a so-called nonpartisan election, in which pretty much anybody with enough petition signatures can run, but Halliby was likely to pull votes from Malling.

I said, "So the mayor will replace Spurlark, either now or after the election, and if Chester Malling is elected, he'll replace Spurlark to show he's doing something proactive."

"And to have his own man in the office. When you appoint a superintendent, he's beholden to you."

"So what does this have to do with you? Wait. I know. One of the top cops wants to be superintendent, and he figures there'll be a new one chosen soon, and whoever it is thinks you're his main competitor?"

"Got it in one."

They'd be right, too. McCoo would be a very serious competitor. He was not in the very top echelon of cops, the deputy superintendents, but there were only five people ranked above him. One of course was the superintendent. Just below him were the four deputy superintendents, each of whom headed up three or four divisions. As chief of the

Detective Division, McCoo was in the next level down. He was, however, the best-known and most-liked top cop. He was at the "Dick Tracy" desk. He'd solved several media-hot cases. And because he always gave credit to the detectives in the field—didn't claim to have solved every case personally, even though it was frequently his experience and insight that had made the difference—the troops liked him and the press corps liked him. You can say all the bad things you want about the press; the fact remains that they are very good at telling a grandstander apart from a guy who really does his job.

Yes, McCoo was popular in the city of Chicago. Yes, he could be a good candidate for superintendent. It would take a serious scandal to discredit him.

An intermittent leak would work better than one big crisis to discredit him. It made a mystery out of the event, and kept building public interest. It was the Nixon effect. If Nixon hadn't tried to cover up, if he'd said at the beginning, "Gee, some of my supporters made a horrible mistake," the story might have peaked and died.

The attack on McCoo seemed well orchestrated.

What was sad was for McCoo, of all people, to get swept into a nasty political wrangle. He loved the job he did, loved detection and the detectives and working the cases. He was a hands-on chief of detectives, not a desk man. I doubt if he wanted to change jobs.

"Want to be superintendent?" I asked.

"Oh, hell, no! The job is just constant crap. Political maneuverings. Stupid banquets. *Conferences!* I hate that stuff. I'm a cop, not a glitterati."

"I think the singular is probably 'glitteratus.' So who do you think is doing this to you?"

"One of the top cops, Cat."

"Such as?"

"One of the deputy superintendents."

"So let's make a list."

"What good will that do?"

"Humor me."

"Greg Winter. Bob Cleary. Paul Bannister. Louise Montoya. People I was in the academy with. People I've known all my working life."

I watched his face. His sadness hurt me. I said, "Or Superintendent Spurlark."

"Spurlark? No way. This makes him look bad."

"No, not necessarily. The Daniello thing makes the CPD look bad already. But it happened. He can't change that. If he focuses the public on a scapegoat, he could fire the scapegoat and get out from under."

"I think that's reaching, Cat."

"Have it your way. But bear one thing in mind: At this point, Spurlark has nothing to lose."

"That's true." There was another gray pause.

"So, McCoo, what now? I'd do anything I could to help you. But exactly what *can* I do? Suppose I wrote a piece explaining the truth, whatever the truth may be?"

"It'd be just another story in a big avalanche of stories."

"How about this? Let me look at the facts of the Jurack case. At the very least," I said, "I'll have a different point of view from you."

Another sad pause.

"So that I'll know the background, you have Bramble make me copies of Shelly Daniello's report and the other data—the autopsy protocol and the lab results, whatever."

"I shouldn't let those out."

"You know me, McCoo. I'm a graveyard. I don't even tell people what the weather's like."

"It'll take her a while."

"So? Then, next, I want to interview the deputy superintendents."

"Oh, good thinking, Cat. Ask them if they're trying to stab me in the back?"

"No, no. I'll do profiles on them. It makes newspaper sense right now. There's a scandal. There's rumor of a change. It's timely for a paper—or maybe my buddies at Channel Three, even—to profile the likely candidates for next superintendent."

I sipped the horrid coffee to give him a few seconds to get used to the idea.

"Cat, cops hate reporters. Cops will tell a reporter *less* than they tell other cops, not more."

"Not true."

"Of course it is. Everybody knows our famous thin blue line mentality—"

"But I'm saying—"

"Just listen for a second without talking so much!"

"Oh, yes, sir! Aye, aye, boss."

"Sorry. Cat, I'm really sorry." He rubbed his forehead. "I realize you're trying to help me."

"Hey, no prob."

"But I'm still right."

"Listen. They'll want to talk right now, much more than they usually would, because they're all running for election now, so to speak."

"I admit there's a window of opportunity here."

"Plus, it's not entirely true cops will tell me less than they'd tell another cop. They'll be more guarded with me. No doubt about it. But they'll talk, most of them. They may not tell me *more*, but they'll tell me *different*."

"Well, that's all very well, but if they're guarded, how is that going to help you?"

"When I interview people, I try to home in on whatever I think they're trying not to say."

"Of course. But these guys are pros. They won't give it up just because you're the greatest reporter in the entire world."

"Yeah, sure. But I'll get an idea of what they don't want to talk about. What they shy away from. Next, I let them run on at length about whatever they will talk about. And that's going to be—"

"Whatever they're proud of. Or whatever they want to sell you."

"Right. So now I've got what they're hiding and what they're selling about themselves. Bear in mind also that there are things I can ask them that you couldn't, because you ought to *know*. So I can ask dumb questions. Then I employ a little study of their body language and how they handle themselves for an idea of their personality type—"

"Sure. As if I shouldn't already know them all the way through."

"Do you?"

He sighed and looked out the window. "I certainly thought I did. I'm obviously wrong about one of them."

"Well, so I guess any second person's opinion is a good corrective."

"I'm beginning to think you may be more accurate in half an hour of observation than I've been after twenty years of knowing these guys."

"Oh, please! Excessive humility does *not* become you, McCoo."

He smiled a very lukewarm smile. "I notice you don't complain about excessive compliments to yourself."

It was upsetting to find McCoo so gloomy. He was no naive child. He knew the press was a voracious mulch machine and did not care what happened later to the people involved, as long as it got its stories. And he was well aware of top-cop backbiting, power struggles, all the effects of the me-first climb up the ladder. But the fact remained that he had worked with the deputy supers all his adult life. He had been in the academy with two of them, Spurlark and Bob Cleary. One, Paul Bannister, had been a sort of mentor to him. He himself had been a mentor to another, Louise Montoya. They weren't just faceless political rivals.

He was too close to it, I thought.

For that matter, this particular incident went well beyond maneuvering for power. This was truly nasty.

Sure, it would be enough to make him sick.

"Come on," I chirped. "It'll be noninvasive, at least." Wait a second, I thought. I'm not really sure about this myself. But it was too late. Just looking at him, I knew he was going to cave in.

When I closed the door of McCoo's office behind me, I was back in the outer office, with his staff. Every one of them swiveled and stared at me, except for Fred Koy, whose desk was behind me on the farther side of the room, so he didn't need to swivel, he just stared. Every eye in the place, eight of them, focused on me.

I said, "Uh—if you're hoping I'll tell you I worked a miracle, I didn't."

Bramble said, "Damn! Yeah, I had hopes."

"But I am going to do some consulting."

"I guess that's good."

Now, Bramble and I had a tense relationship when we first met several years ago. She is a tall, wiry black woman of thirty-five or forty. An eleven-year veteran of the Chicago police force, she's been McCoo's secretary for at least five. When she first saw me she assumed I was a reporter hanging around her boss in order to surprise or wheedle him into a hasty statement, get some confidential material and then print it—slightly exaggerated—and make a big name for myself. Well, he wouldn't and I wouldn't and now she knows it. Her attitude has become almost welcoming over the years.

The fact that she had turned to me for help when all else had failed was a real vote of confidence. And expressing it was a real act of humility. I was touched, but knew that she wouldn't appreciate my saying so.

"He was actually drinking the instant coffee," I said, "until it spilled." They all groaned.

Bramble said, "That's bad."

Koy said, "Very bad."

Tracy Shoemaker said, "Yesterday too."

Fred Koy said, "We've just got to be patient. And strong. It'll blow over."

"Yeah, like a hurricane blows over," Bramble said. "Leaves piles of shit in its wake." She stirred the mail and papers on her desk. There were a large batch of letters, some padded envelopes, the top one reading "Court Tapes, Do Not Crush," and under it all a fresh newspaper. She pushed the newspaper into view. "See?"

CITY TO PROBE SHOOTING, said the headline.

Bramble read aloud. " 'Alderman Rhonda Barrington-Bloom is calling for a probe into the actions taken by the Chicago Police Department following the shooting of one police officer by another.' " Now Bramble switched to a whining tone. " ' "I am not advocating an independent inquiry into the shooting itself, unless the reconvened round table fails to produce results," ' Bloom said at the City News Bureau today, ' "but I am demanding a probe into hiring practices and review practices of the Chicago Police Department. It is possible that Officer Jurack should have been terminated years ago and that department investigators are keeping that aspect of the case from the public."

" 'Bloom's remarks came today, just after this reporter revealed that a confidential department study of Jurack's record showed many instances of citizen complaints. It was not clear whether Chief of Detectives Harold McCoo considers this material relevant to the inquiry. McCoo could not be reached for comment—' "

Bramble hurled the paper at the file cabinet and shouted, "What a load of crap!"

I said, "It doesn't even make sense. If Jurack was an abusive cop, that should fortify Daniello's story. They're being inconsistent."

"Are newspapers supposed to be consistent?" Bramble asked.

"Uh, no."

Fred said, "Trouble is, that kind of crap lasts. Mud sticks." He got to his feet. "You wanted us to deliver those files," he said to Bramble.

"Right. Make sure you explain our criteria to them," she said. To me, she added, "Not connected to the Daniello case, but it's getting so I feel we have to explain every damn thing that anybody could possibly misunderstand."

Russell got up too, collecting a manila file folder.

"We'll ride down with you, if you're leaving, Cat," he said. "Fred and I have to go to Area Six with some papers."

Bramble said, "McCoo's life in the department is never going to be the same. I mean, up to now he's always been their fair-haired boy, if you'll pardon the expression."

Tracy Shoemaker said, "Cat, there *has* to be something you can do."

"Look, you can't put back the clock," I said. "But I'm going to go see an editor about a story. If we can get to the bottom of what's going on, we'll have one advantage going for us. The public has got itself whipped into a frenzy over this, and that's not all bad. The hardest thing is getting them interested in an injustice in the first place. This way we don't have to set the express train in motion. We just have to deflect it."

• 4 •

The morning was bright and breezy when I stepped out of the CPD onto the street. It was sixty-five degrees, warm at this hour for mid-March. A good day for walking. Walking would keep me from falling asleep. At least I hoped so; falling asleep in the intersection of Monroe and Michigan Avenue would amount to falling asleep forever.

I figured to hike quickly to the north Loop, to the *Chicago Today* building, a landmark with masonry walls six feet thick at the base, similar to the famous Monadnock. While I walked, I would think up a way to sell my editor Hal Briskman on the idea of profiling the top cops. Hal would ask why. Good question. We certainly couldn't say that we were trying to find out who was sabotaging Harold McCoo. We didn't even want anybody to see the connection. We couldn't say we were doing the piece because a new mayor might get rid of Spurlark and there might be a new man at the top, plus a shake-up in the top ranks. You didn't say that kind of thing. Or at least not in a descriptive article. That kind of pontification was for one of our three political columnists, Ms. J. Q. Pundit, Mr. I. M. Acerbic, or Mr. Just-Folks-Like-You.

So what sort of approach?

"The CPD—a Half-Billion-Dollar Company—Who Runs It?" Too long but not a totally bad idea.

"What Makes Chicago's Police Department Different?" Well, sure, but different from what? And why ask the question?

"The CPD Enters the 21st Century." Hmmm. Maybe there was a germ of an idea there. Certainly the current top cops were the people who would take the department into the year 2000.

One thing you could always be sure of. If Hal Briskman thought it was an idea, then it was an idea.

"Cat, you look sick."

"Well, then look at something else, dammit!"

"Whooo!" Hal said. "Did we get up on the wrong side of our bed this morning?"

"We got up on the wrong side of our bed thirty-two hours ago, and we haven't been in bed since! Oh, I'm sorry, Hal. I'm just touchy. I'm a little freaked out about this Jurack shooting."

I saw comprehension pass over his face. Hal was mentally putting my friendship with McCoo, of which he was aware, together with McCoo's recent lambasting in the press, including Hal's paper.

The offices of *Chicago Today* were quiet and clean. Not like the old days when people actually used typewriters. Now the muted *pat-pat* of keyboards was the only sound. Except for the occasional shrieked curse, of course, or the trilling of telephones.

"I want to do a story on the deputy superintendents and superintendent, Hal."

"The top echelon of the police department? Why? Put it another way, *you* might want to, but why do I want to?"

"Uh—it seems like a good time. You know, the year 2000 is coming. Who's going to take us into the twenty-first century?"

"Why do we care?"

"Because we're public-spirited."

"Oh, please. People don't read the paper to become better citizens. I occasionally hope that keeping up with events will *make* them better citizens, but, hey, I'm an optimist."

"Uh-huh. Like Geraldo is reclusive. Well, there's likely to be a top-cop shake-up. No matter which way the mayoral election goes."

"Cat." He put his hands on my shoulders and looked in my eyes. "Level with me."

My defenses were down. I couldn't think of a good lie, so I told the truth. "I want to find out who's behind the attack on McCoo."

"I thought so. I suppose you believe he's dealing straight with the Jurack killing?"

"McCoo's always straight. In a devious world, he's always honest. Maybe that's why people don't always love him. But they respect him."

"Let me change the question a little: Do you think the Jurack killing went down the way the woman cop, uh, Shelly Daniello, said it did?"

"I don't know. I haven't looked at the case. But if McCoo thinks it did, it did. He's incorruptible."

"That isn't what some people are saying."

"Including one of your underpaid, underinformed columnists."

"Mm-mmm. We don't white-glove people just because they're your friends, Cat. You know, it's also possible McCoo could be totally honest but wrong."

"McCoo isn't only honest, he's canny. If the shooting makes sense to him the way Shelly Daniello told it, then that's the way it happened. Somebody's out to get him, Hal. He looked good to be the next superintendent, and somebody didn't want that."

"Nobody is infallible."

"All right, all right. As near as I can tell you, McCoo believes Shelly Daniello is an honest person. He could be mistaken about that, but he's a good judge of people and he has her record to go by, too. It could also be that Daniello herself is honestly mistaken for some reason none of us understands yet."

"Maybe."

"So what about my story?"

Hal said, "Let's see. How about—mmm—'Who Are the

Top Cops?' We could just ask that question, flat out. I like
that. It's simple. It's clean."

"It doesn't explain why we're doing the story."

"I like that, too. People can take it the way they want:
either they'll think that from this group a new superintendent
will be selected, or that these people's hiring practices permitted a trigger-happy woman cop to stay on the job, or by
ignoring the signs of abuse failed to stop a cop from abusing
his wife, whatever. Something for everybody."

"A Rorschach of an article?" But it could be interesting to a
lot of people for a lot of reasons. What did I care? I had what
I wanted, or rather what McCoo wanted. "Is my friendship
with McCoo likely to affect what they tell me?"

"Doubt it. I don't think anybody is aware the two of you are
more than occasional interviewer-interviewee. As far as I can
remember, you've never even quoted him in print."

"I guess. He never wanted to be quoted. I haven't bruited
our friendship about in the journalism business. He's mine,
not everybody's."

"Plus, you're known but you're not famous."

"Thanks a lot."

"Fifteen hundred words, okay?"

"I can't even order a sandwich in fifteen hundred words."

"That's all I'm paying for. Next: Don't forget I'm expecting
your article on the paramedics."

I agreed and left, tired but happy enough.

I marched along the hallway, my heels clicking. The
elderly building was floored with that old kind of ceramic
tile—small hexagons, about an inch across, in black and
white. Those things never wear out! They were installed here
in the late 1800s, and after more than a century of shoes passing over them, decades and decades of changing styles of
shoes and boots and winter galoshes, mud and snow and ice
and salt, these days probably Rollerblades, they don't even
look worn. Ten years ago I was really tired of them, but now
they're becoming sort of a sign of stability in a world of too

much entropy. Much better than that plastic stuff in police
headquarters. Economical—install it once and it's good for a
hundred years.

Somebody said, "Cat!"

A tall, slender woman carrying a briefcase was silhouetted
against the light from the far street doors.

"Cat! McCoo said I'd find you here."

"Bramble?"

· 5 ·

"I thought I'd save you the walk back," she said. "And besides, I had to go out to lunch in an hour anyway . . ."

She hesitated and a look of annoyance came over her face. "I have to stop doing that," she said. "I'm taking assertiveness training. I'm on a tell-it-like-it-is program." My mouth fell open. Bramble—not assertive enough? But I shut up smartly and let her go on. "I did not come over here to save you the walk. I came over here because I couldn't stand it in the office any longer."

"I'm not surprised. I've never seen him like that."

"What it is . . . is this particular bunch of deputy superintendents are people he really likes. It isn't always that way. Our last big enchilada wanted to appoint wallpaper deputies wherever he could get away with it."

"Wallpaper?"

"Oh, you know. Hangs around, looks good, doesn't *do* anything."

I chuckled. "You mentioned lunch. I know a place a block from here with the best food in Chicago—"

"Child, you do know how to talk."

Hermione's Heaven truly is the best place to eat in Chicago. Hermione herself is a queen-sized woman who is not patient with the word "diet." Or people who want to bug her about her weight. Today she was wearing a scarlet caftan and scarlet turban. I said, "Wow!"

"I call it the walking-fireplug look," she said.

Bramble shook her head in admiration, muttering, "My, my. Strong, very strong."

"One more minute and you wouldn't have been able to get a table," Hermione said.

Bramble said, "It's eleven-fifteen!"

"Around here the rush starts at eleven." And she was right. There were now several people standing behind us in the entranceway. "Today's specials are 'corned beef and cabbage and corned beef and cabbage and corned beef and cabbage,' which basically is a whole lot of corned beef and cabbage, or my 'ribs and bibs.' My barbecued ribs are in real barbecue sauce—molasses and spices, not that bastardized tomato sauce. And today you're in luck; an old favorite returns. Chocolate cheesecake, topped with crystallized orange."

Bramble said, "Oh, my *dear!*"

We went for the corned beef and cabbage, not ribs, because we wanted to be able to handle papers at the table.

I said, "Uh, Bramble? You're taking assertiveness training? I can't believe you ever needed a program like that."

"Think I'm too outspoken?"

"Uh—well—I wouldn't say 'too.' I'd say 'enough.' "

"I wasn't with my family. Family is different. Probably always have been outspoken on the job. For that matter, maybe I wanted to be a cop because it let me be different. Let me take charge."

"You surely used to be frank enough that you didn't like me."

"Didn't trust you. Different thing entirely. Now I do. The boss always did. He's got a real talent for judging human beings, you know. Which is one of the reasons I think he's so impacted by this leak."

"I can understand that. And I'm glad you sent for me."

"I'm glad too. I hope."

The corned beef arrived, on platters the size of a California surfboard. Hermione did not short the customer by piling on lots of cabbage and a little roof of corned beef. The meat stretched pinkly from one end of the plate to the other and hung half an inch off the sides.

"Mmm-mm," I said.

"That's the right word. Now, speaking of judging people, I've got Shelly Daniello's work history. And her incident report. And a transcript of the round table. McCoo says her story rings true. Me, I can't tell. If somebody'd been beating on my sister, and I had a chance to shoot him under circumstances that *looked* good, would I do it?"

"You asking me?"

"Right. Tell me yes or no. Don't waffle."

So I looked at her. After a few seconds I said, "Ye-es. You would."

"But?"

"But I didn't say *where* you'd shoot him."

She laughed and pushed the Daniello papers to me. On top was the incident report Daniello had filed that day, at the end of her tour.

"Bramble, do they go out of their way to teach police officers how not to write anything in normal language?"

"We're an in-group, Marsala. We have our own lingo, and we love it. You wouldn't understand. It's a cop thing."

Daniello's bald account seemed an inadequate way to summarize an event that took one life and looked as if it would destroy several careers. And there was no hint of the depression and terror of a brutal marriage. Of course that really wasn't fair. This wasn't the place for it. Plus, Shelly Daniello had spent years in pain over her sister's marriage. She had probably tried to help all three Juracks, the child included. Now look what had happened.

I glanced at the other sheets while we ate. There were several pages of reports from supervisory cops, and a lab report and an autopsy protocol.

I said, "Can I keep these?"

"Yes. All these copies are yours. But listen, you've got to

CONTINUATION OF NARRATIVE

At 1531 hours 3-7-97 responding officer and partner responded to a call to a domestic violence at 1764 Barcourt. Upon arrival, r/o discovered the husband, Ben Jurack engaged in committing battery upon the body of his wife, Marie Jurack, who was screaming that she had been stabbed. R/o cautioned Jurack to drop the knife, but despite additional cautions he continued to threaten Mrs. Jurack. He then lunged toward Mrs. Jurack and r/o with the knife. R/o shouted "stop" to no avail. Fearing for my life and the safety of my partner, and of the victim Mrs. Jurack, I discharged my weapon, striking Jurack in the lower chest or upper abdomen. R/o's partner entered the room at that moment and radioed immediately for an ambulance. Subj. was pronounced dead at University Hospital. Investigating officers were called and premises placed under seal. Scene was transferred to control of investigating officers from Area 3.

FOR USE BY BUREAU OF INVESTIGATIVE SERVICES ONLY

I HAVE REVIEWED THIS REPORT AND BY MY SIGNATURE INDICATE THAT IT IS ACCEPTABLE.

SUPERVISOR'S SIGNATURE   DATE (DAY MO YR)

SUPV. STAR NO. 9 7 7 1 2

POSTMORTEM REPORT   DEPARTMENT OF HEALTH   CASE NO.   PAGE

                                 COOK COUNTY   723-96   2 of 5

                                 2121 W. HARRISON

                                 CHICAGO IL 60612

This forty-seven year old, well-developed, well-nourished white male weighs approximately 205 pounds and is approximately 72" in length.

GENERAL

The body is received wearing a white armless undershirt with low neck. The shirt is pushed up to the upper torso and is heavily stained with blood on both the anterior and posterior aspects. The body is wearing blue wool trousers and green plaid boxer shorts. It is wearing black socks and black leather-like shoes.

EXTERNAL EXAMINATION

The hair is straight and dark brown. The irides are green with pupils regular, round and equal at .5 cm diameter. The teeth are in a neglected state of repair, and there is a partial upper plate. The mouth is otherwise not unusual. The external nares are not unusual. The external auditory canals are not unusual. The trachea is in the midline. There is a round wound directly over the Xiphoid process from which a small amount of red fluid exudes. The chest is not otherwise unusual. The external genitalia are not unusual. There is a small amount of blood on the back of the right hand, which is not associated with any underlying injuries. The knuckles are reddened but the skin is not broken. The extremities are not otherwise unusual. The posterior is not unusual with the exception of a large irregularly shaped wound lying 2 cm to the left of C6.

EXTERNAL EVIDENCE OF INJURY

1. Above the left eye there is a well-defined purple area associated with a slight swelling .5-1.0 cm wide and 3 cm long, which begins 3 cm above the orbital margin at the distal edge of the frontal eminence.

2. A circular wound 2 cm in diameter lies directly over the

Emmy Suvitha, M.D.

[ALL PAGES MUST BE SIGNED]

MK-050-C

realize that you're not supposed to have them. You can't quote from them in writing."

"I wouldn't!"

"I accept that. But you can't let anybody else know you've seen them. Even your editor. You'll have to keep them in a safe place at home where nobody else can stumble on them. You're media, and if anybody knew you had them, it could look to an outsider as if McCoo was using you to run his own media leak to the press. That's absolutely the last thing we need now."

"Well, it won't happen."

"And speaking of the leaks, the boss says you're going to talk with the top cops."

"Yes."

"Bear in mind that even though they could request the lab reports and autopsy and so on, that material doesn't go to them automatically. Reports of an incident go to the area commander in charge of the investigation and from there up to McCoo. If any of the deputy superintendents wanted them, they'd have to ask for them. The superintendent is entitled to them, naturally, and so is Bannister. He's McCoo's boss. But they don't just get sent data on active cases automatically. They have to request them. And I have no record that they did—until it blew up into a huge scandal."

"What about the area commander, then? Could he be the source of the leak?" There are six area headquarters in Chicago, geographically spaced out, located in certain of the twenty-five district police stations. Patrol officers work out of the districts. Detectives work out of areas, and each district and area has its own commander. The local area commander would collect a lot of the Jurack data for McCoo.

"Possibly. But an area commander is too far down on the totem pole to be a candidate for the next superintendent, unless he's some kind of superstar. And Ainslie isn't. He's just a good, old-line cop. So why should he risk his neck?"

"Maybe to curry favor with somebody who might be the next superintendent."

"Hey, that's actually a surprisingly good idea, Cat!"

"Thanks a lot," I said. "Don't fall all over yourself being amazed."

"I didn't mean—"

"Don't sweat it."

"But that explanation doesn't really work. A couple of things have been leaked that have only been in our office. They didn't go up through the area structure at all."

"Too bad. Such as?"

"Jurack's work history, for example. He worked in the Eighteenth District, and his record came from Personnel. The Eighteenth District is Area Three. His record had been in our office for several days. Plus, we had a spousal-abuse study done out of our office, and parts of that were leaked. It was a study the department commissioned from an independent social-statistics research organization, and it was completed three months ago. So it had been available for quite some time."

"Oh."

"I had an idea yesterday about the pattern of the leaks. Now that we've had ten days of this, I'm beginning to chart just when each leak came out in the press. So I can guess when the data actually leaked. That's assuming you news people use hot copy the instant you get it. Do you?"

"If it's hot, definitely. It would be in the next possible issue. There's no sense sitting on it. Somebody else might break the news ahead of you."

"That's what I thought."

"Well, what are you finding out?"

"Let me get it straight first. If it's what it seems, it isn't going to make McCoo very happy."

"He's not very happy already."

"You got *that* right. I've never seen him like this. Even when Susanne was sick."

I said, "No. When that happened, he was mad." Susanne, McCoo's wife, had had breast cancer a year earlier.

"Furious."

"And brave, too. He's such a good guy. He was really supportive to her."

"This is too depressing to talk about," Bramble said, rubbing her eyes. "Did somebody mention the words 'chocolate cheesecake'?"

"Yes. Gonna have some? I think under the circumstances, I really deserve a piece, too."

"It's the stress. Stress increases the minimum daily requirement of chocolate."

When the dessert arrived, Bramble slowly swallowed a large forkful and smiled. "See. I'm better already."

"Hermione surely knows her chocolate."

"Even this crystallized orange on top isn't bad. Normally I don't like candied fruit. I had a boyfriend three or four years back who used to travel for a hardware firm. Atlantic Seaboard mostly. He used to send me trays of candied fruit from Florida. Stuffed dates and candied pineapple, maraschino cherries, figs wrapped in red and green foil and little white plastic forks to stab them with. I'd never get one of the damn things without wishing it was chocolate and having to tell him thanks, whether I liked it or not."

"So what happened? You broke up?"

"Oh, not because of the fruit. Other problems. But I never could make him understand. I mean, just because you wrap a fig in foil doesn't make it chocolate."

I got home at 3 P.M. When I walked in the door, I found Long John Silver perched on the bedroom lampshade. Long John does not like to have his schedule disrupted and he had already told me several times that my staying out all night upset him. He squawked, "Prophet said I! Thing of evil!" Usually he quotes Shakespeare, and right now I would have preferred it.

I left a message on Teddy's machine. "If Mom wants to do dinner Sunday, it's okay with me."

Then I sat down and held my head with both hands. I had been awake over thirty-five hours. At the age of sixteen, or even twenty-six, I wouldn't have minded the loss of sleep. But by the time you're in your mid-thirties, pulling an all-nighter has lost its luster. I'd go straight to bed.

Oh, no! Hal had said I had to finish the paramedic article by tomorrow morning. And I'd better do it. I needed the money. Blast!

· 6 ·

"You just sit. I'm making coffee," I told McCoo. "No more instant for you."

"Thank you, Cat," he said, in a dreary, polite, bland voice that broke my heart. Since when was McCoo either polite or bland? Crabby, maybe. Demanding, maybe. And a lot more sensitive to people's feelings than he might appear. But not polite, not Wonder Bread plain polite.

It was Wednesday morning. I had handed in the EMT story, thank goodness, and got it out of the way, although usually I like to let a story sit cooling off for a couple of days and then recheck it to see if there are ugly lumps that need ironing. But I didn't have time on this one. Sending a piece out there raw made me uneasy, but friendship was more important than career right now.

McCoo's coffee grinder stood ready. There were three different bags of coffee beans. I picked the Sumatra mandheling. What did I know? If he had bought it, it was going to be good.

It smelled great grinding. It smelled great brewing. It smelled great pouring into cups. It smelled so great Bramble stuck her head in the door, saying to McCoo, "I could pretend to need your signature on some formset, but . . ." and she sniffed the air meaningfully. I poured her a cup and she sat down.

I handed a cup to McCoo. He sipped.

"Not bad, Marsala," he said. "But not perfect. Not quite strong enough. Listen up, now. A little more coffee in the pot next time. You shouldn't be able to see the bottom of the cup, you got that part right, but you also shouldn't be able to see the sides."

"McCoo! You're fussy. You're critical. You're back."

"Fooled you."

Bramble said, "I think I'll take this up with the Fraternal Order of Police. Playing mind games with the help isn't permitted." But she was smiling happily.

"Well, I'm not really playing mind games," he said. "I'm still appalled that anybody would hurt the department just for a shot at being superintendent. But this morning I woke up totally sick of being depressed by it. I'm good and mad. It's time to fight back."

I got a container of real cream from his mini-refrigerator. We all took some. There are times for avoiding fat and calories. This was not one of them.

"I've been over the papers Bramble gave me," I said. "The lab report is unequivocal that there was powder stippling on Jurack's undershirt. That shirt was near the muzzle of her gun. If Shelly Daniello says she fired from three or four feet, either she doesn't remember accurately, or she's lying."

Bramble said to McCoo, "It was a stress situation, boss. She may not remember clearly."

"That's not an excuse," McCoo said. "It's part of her job to remember clearly in stressful situations. Cops have to give testimony in court about the behavior of defendants. Even when the defendant has been shooting at them. They're supposed to do it accurately."

"Plus," I said, "Daniello claims that she didn't shoot Jurack in the presence of his child, but that doesn't seem to hold up. Her partner Hubner gave the round table a clear statement that when he ran into the room, Daniello had just shot Jurack, and the child was cowering in the corner, not near enough to the door to have run in *after* her father was shot."

"I know."

"And the third discrepancy, that bruise on Jurack's head. She could have hit him, you know."

"Shelly Daniello isn't that kind of officer," McCoo said. "She's got a good, solid record. She's put in her time in active districts and she's had far less than the average number of citizen complaints. Nothing is a hundred percent, and I don't know her very well, but you get a sense about police officers when you're been around as long as I have."

"This was her own family, McCoo. The emotions are stronger. It's an entirely different situation."

"I don't believe she executed him."

"You seem awfully sure about a person you hardly know."

"There's background."

"You'd better tell me."

"About four years ago, in February, Daniello was on routine patrol as a ninety-nine unit."

"One-person car."

"Right. It was maybe two A.M. She had an on-view, saw two men struggling at the end of the Michigan Avenue Bridge. You know, where—"

"The bridge that suddenly flipped up last year."

"Right. She saw one man pick up a rock or a chunk of paving stone and strike the other man on the head several times. She leaped out of her squad car, ran down the offender and handcuffed him, called for an ambulance for the other man. All the right things. The injured man died. That made it homicide. The ASA wanted the rock, but nobody could find it. We sent detectives and evidence techs over in daylight, and they looked through the snow and slush, but they couldn't find it either. The ASA was upset. Her commander was furious. Said she either should have found it or maybe her story wasn't accurate. She swore it was. She said it was a rock about the size of a softball and the assailant had tossed it onto the sidewalk when he saw her get out of the squad car."

"Maybe it rolled into the river."

"See, that's the thing. She said it hadn't. But she could so easily have said it did, and saved herself the trouble."

"So what happened?"

"It didn't make sense to me. I wandered over there the next afternoon. The snow had melted, so I figured if there was a rock, I'd find it. No rock. But I saw some hair and dried tissue on the pavement, partly protected by a mailbox. You see what had happened?"

"Uh—"

"The hair and tissue matched the victim. It was ten feet from the place the struggle happened. You can't throw hair ten feet. Shelly Daniello was right. The victim had been hit by a softball-sized chunk of ice."

"Oh."

"And she could so easily have gotten free of criticism just by saying the rock rolled into the river."

"Okay. Let's say Shelly is truthful. Could this be a setup?"

"Setup how?"

"Somebody chooses Shelly Daniello as a patsy. Somehow they get Jurack riled up so he beats his wife—give him a hard time at work, maybe—knowing Daniello would be called to the scene. She has to do something to stop him from killing his wife. And they've arranged for her partner Hubner to lie about it."

"It would take a lot of arranging."

"One person in the district, maybe his sergeant, plus Hubner."

"Why do it?"

"In order to get at you."

"That's really reaching, Cat. Hubner could lose his job."

"There's such a thing as payoffs."

"Not enough money in it. Even the superintendent doesn't make enough to pay off Brad Hubner for the rest of his life. Anyhow, how would they know she'd kill him?"

"Hoped. They could always try again with somebody else if it didn't work."

"How would they know it would make me personally look bad?"

"Oh, that's easy. They just have to slant what they leak to the papers. There are always several ways to report any news." I sighed. "Look, we can come back to this later. Let's take another tack. We know the autopsy results about that bruise on Jurack's head got leaked. Is there a possibility the fact was leaked from the Medical Examiner's Office, not your office here?"

"Of course," McCoo said. "Anybody can talk, even the ME. But the ME didn't have the lab results on the powder burns on the shirt. That testing was done here in the CPD lab. And he didn't have Hubner's testimony. That came out of the round table inquiry. So the ME couldn't have done it alone. And the CPD lab couldn't have done it alone. And don't even try to convince me that there's some megaconspiracy involving techs and doctors and cops and what-all just to get me. That's too stupid and Byzantine. I'd just as soon believe the Sewer Rats got together with the Tunnel People to bring down the CPD."

I loved it when McCoo sounded like himself. I said, "Okay. Give me some nuts and bolts here. What form are your files in?"

"Paper and cyberspace," Bramble said. "And certain ones are only paper and certain ones are only on computer."

"And data has been read from both?"

"Yup."

"On these cyberfiles, is there automatically a notation of who has read them?"

"If anybody other than me and Bramble reads a file—say the superintendent reads it from his office terminal, which he can if the material is entered on certain files—a code number appears on the file."

"And there isn't any?"

"Nope. And very few even have access," McCoo said.

"Even within your office?"

"This was sensitive stuff. Bramble filed it. We don't exactly keep secrets in the office, but we're discreet."

"McCoo, some of those newspaper accounts were so detailed, you'd think they had a Xerox of your files."

"I know."

"Several people in the department must have asked for the documents legitimately. There's been a lot of media attention."

"Well, not as many requests for the actual paper as you might think," McCoo said. "We gave a verbal report at first to the News Affairs Office so they could talk to the press. I briefed Nolly Johnson myself. My verbal report didn't include the head bruise or the powder burns. There'd be no reason to give that to the press at such an early stage of the investigation, plus we needed to keep certain data to ourselves if we were ever going to try to catch one of the principals in a lie. The press has pretty well screwed that up now. The round table board of inquiry had Daniello's and Hubner's account of the incident by the day after the shooting, but neither the lab report nor the autopsy results were in by then. And we've been giving short verbal reports to the superintendent at intervals."

"What about the IAD?"

"Oh, Internal Affairs got everything we had. But first we received it here from the lab or the ME, then we duplicated it, then we messengered it to them. So sometimes they got it a day or two *after* it had appeared in the newspapers."

"Oh. They must have been thrilled, coming in second."

McCoo said, "It had to be somebody who could come in here and take what he wanted, maybe run it off on our Xerox."

"And knew where to look."

"Yes, and knew where to look. And what to look for."

"And had a key to get in."

"A top cop," McCoo said.

"Or an ADS."

An assistant deputy superintendent was a sort of aide, a high-level facilitator for a deputy superintendent. McCoo said, "An ADS wouldn't have anything to gain."

"Oh, not for himself; he wouldn't be in line for superintendent. He'd have something to gain from his boss, though, if the boss got him to do the dirty work."

Bramble said, "From his boss, he could get a promotion. And if his boss became the next superintendent, the sky's the limit."

"Or," I said, "he could blackmail his boss for the rest of the man's career."

McCoo said, "Well, that's the downside. You always take a risk if you get somebody to do your dirty work for you. If that's what happened, somebody wants it very badly."

Bramble said grimly, "Everybody wants it badly."

I said, "All right, let's talk about the real possibilities. The best candidate for traitor is Bob Cleary. He's first deputy, so he'd step in automatically if the superintendent were disabled or died."

"Absolutely not Bob!" McCoo barked.

"Why not?"

"Bob is not a rat. Bob would never do anything to hurt the department. He's from a cop family. He's the third generation of his family to be a Chicago cop. His grandfather walked a beat in Back-of-the-Yards in the days of nightsticks and little call boxes on light poles. His father was a district commander. Bob has a brother who's a detective and his daughter is a cop in Narcotics."

"Well, I hate to say it, McCoo, but that doesn't make him a saint. Wasn't there a third-generation Chicago cop last year who was receiving stolen property at a warehouse on the northwest side, out near O'Hare? I covered part of the story myself. Had such a big operation he needed six panel trucks? Got caught because he forgot to update his city stickers and a cop stopped him and got to wondering why the van was full of electronic gear when it was labeled 'It's a Dog's Life—Pet Boarding and Grooming.' "

"Yeah. Well, it happens. But not Bob. Bob and I were in the academy together. We've been friends for thirty-five years. He and his wife and Susanne and I go out once a month and do dinner in Greektown. I'm his daughter's godfather."

"All right! All right. Forget Cleary. Let's move on. What about Gregory Dennison Winter?"

He was thoughtful. "I don't believe so. He thinks too highly of himself."

"Oh?"

"Everything has always come easy to Winter. He went to law school, aced it, had the perfect brain for it. Said it was easy. Then, he says, he wanted to do something different from the rest of his family. They're all lawyers or corporation CEOs. He came on the cops and had a big case right out of the box. Got promoted. Had connections. Zoomed right on up. To be fair to him, he's real good at his job because he's real smart. To be even fairer, he works hard. But unlike most people, he gets just about everything he works for."

"Maybe he figures he's hit a ceiling and needs to give himself some dishonest help."

"Cat, he's only fifty. With compulsory retirement at sixty-three and superintendents lasting at most three–four years, he knows he has three or four shots at the job before he's done. With his record and connections, he's got to believe it'll fall in his lap someday."

"Doesn't Winter have family money?"

"Yeah, he has."

"He's the one who could make a payoff then, to his ADS to rummage in your files."

"I still don't believe it."

"Paul Bannister, then. He's your direct superior. He might be able to get the data without leaving a trail in the computer. By E-mail, maybe?"

Bramble said, "No, there'd still be a trail. And remember, some of this is paper, not on the computer. Hard copy. He'd have to see it in physical form."

"Well, he could come in here and read it, couldn't he?"

Bramble said, "We sure haven't seen him."

"Anyway," McCoo said, "he's not a good candidate for superintendent. He's sixty-two, and that's too old. Besides, he hasn't been well. He had a heart attack last year that News Affairs glossed over, called it heat exhaustion or some lame thing. But it wasn't. It was a real, full-fledged heart attack."

"He could still hope a new mayor might want him as temporary superintendent, a place-holder while the mayor looks around for his main man."

"That's not the way they work."

"Ever?"

"Well . . ."

"Does Bannister want it?"

"Well, yeah. I guess he wants it. It'd be the capper on a long, distinguished career. But Cat, he knows he doesn't have a chance."

"People have been known to believe they can get what they want—irrationally believe it—if they want it badly enough."

"He's not crazy. I just don't buy it."

"That leaves us with Louise Montoya."

"Oh, not Louise, Cat."

"Why not Louise?"

"Louise Montoya is a tough cookie."

"And that means she can't attack you?"

"That means she'd attack me to my face. Louise is the definition of 'in your face.' She's a west sider. An Hispanic west sider. Used to be a gang girl."

"She was in a gang? What are you saying? You can't mean this is a good thing!"

"She ran with a gang in high school, such as they were back then. I don't think the gangs then were as vicious as they are now, but they weren't Caspar Milquetoast, either. Fewer guns, but more knives. Bicycle chains, razors, like that. Then she realized how stupid it all was. She worked her way through Loyola, but she was supporting her brother at the same time, and it took her six years. She was twenty-six when she graduated. Thought of going to law school. Then she decided the way to serve her community was in the police department. Rocketed up in the department in spite of being extremely outspoken. She made sergeant in three years. She's fifty-three now, and that's young for a deputy superintendent."

"She sounds ambitious. She probably wants to be superintendent."

"Probably? She *definitely* wants to be superintendent. She *intends* to be the first woman superintendent. She's told me so maybe two dozen times. But she wants it her way. Face-to-face. Beat down the competition by her sheer force, determination, brains, will, and tenacity. This is a woman who wouldn't cheat at solitaire, because it would be the same as losing. This woman is *not* a sneak, Cat."

"All right, McCoo. You've just given convincing arguments that none of them could be the saboteur. I guess it all didn't happen. Want me to go home now? I could use the sleep. I could use two whole days of sleep."

"Maybe it's not one of the top cops."

"Nobody else has anything to gain. The other people at your level aren't well-known enough to be superintendent candidates."

"Maybe somebody just hates me."

Bramble said, "Yeah. You've put away a lot of people in twenty-five years."

"But still, the people I've put away wouldn't have access to the reports."

I said, "Convicts have brothers and sisters and children and husbands and wives. And some of them could be cops."

McCoo said, "But that's *really* far-fetched."

"Then it's a top cop."

"Oh, hell, you're right. It's unlikely to be anybody except candidates for superintendent. But I still just can't . . . Greg Winter, Bob Cleary, Paul Bannister, Louise Montoya? Damn!" He held his head with both hands. "Cat, if you can find out which of them is sabotaging me, I'm in your debt forever."

All the top cops had offices in the CPD building. I wanted to see Bob Cleary, because he was the highest-ranking after the superintendent. It turned out he and the rest were in a morning meeting with the superintendent, but Cleary was expected to emerge in thirty minutes. I bet they were discussing the Daniello case and probably talking about McCoo as well.

Cleary's ADS actually thought he would be willing to be interviewed. Amazing! Obviously he was already campaigning for superintendent. One rule of reporting is simple: Strike while the iron is hot. So I told the ADS I'd be back shortly. A maple-frosted doughnut at Mel's wouldn't be bad, and Mel's was only two blocks away, north on State.

The crumbling sidewalks here were a hazard. Especially to a person who writes interview questions in her head while she walks. I stumbled over a jutting piece of concrete, but caught myself before falling. In this area of spotty gentrification, fresh new sidewalk abuts sidewalk that looks as if Chicago had major earthquakes. I stepped over the rubble and went on.

I felt suddenly as if I had tripped again, but I hadn't. The air shifted slightly. Then there was a *crack/whump* sound that hit me from behind.

I whirled around.

For a couple of seconds I thought the sound had been thunder. There was a pattering like raindrops around me.

The drops were tiny pieces of glass. A couple of shards fell in my hair. I shouldn't have turned to look so fast; now there were fragments in my eyelashes. By the time I realized that, the glass had stopped falling. I shook my head to clear my hair and eyes.

A block behind me was the Chicago Police Department. On floors seven and nine, on the side facing the alley, the window glass was shattered. But on the eighth floor the glass was gone and the chicken-wire reinforcement ballooned, bulging and ragged, some of it hanging in tatters.

The eighth floor facing the alley. That was the outer office of Chief of Detectives Harold McCoo.

◇ 7 ◇

I ran. Back to the CPD I ran, making for the wide bank of front doors as fast as I could.

I wasn't fast enough. By the time I lurched out of breath to the center door, three uniformed cops had placed their bodies in front. I nearly collided with the tallest one. "Hold it," he said.

"I have a friend inside."

"Lady, so do we all."

This was so horribly true that my head went back as if slapped. "Was it the eighth floor?" I asked.

"I don't know, lady."

I stepped away and looked up. It *was* the eighth floor, of course, and I already knew it. I was just hoping the cop would say I was wrong. Suddenly I realized I was shaking. "He might be dead," I whispered to myself.

Could I go around the back and sneak in? No, there wasn't any access there. Years ago they'd put inspectors and metal detectors at the front, and closed all the other entrances except the First District Station doors in the back. The First District wouldn't let me go through into the other part of the building while this was happening, any more than these guys in front would.

Standing there useless, unable to help McCoo, I tried to console myself. Think of something good: If McCoo had to be hurt, better he was here than out on the street alone someplace. Everybody in the building was trained in first aid. Everybody knew enough to send for the paramedics at once. If only—if only he was still alive.

What about Bramble? Outspoken, loyal Bramble. Or Fred Koy, Fred the cheerful. Or Tracy Shoemaker? Or Russell Lupinski?

My mind started bargaining with the facts. It can't have been a very *big* bomb, can it? No, definitely not. The wall was undamaged. The wire-reinforced glass was blown outward, but not atomized, and the window frames were intact. Surely that meant it wasn't a huge blast. Surely. Please?

My eyes were clouding. I refused to cry. People would see me. I swiped my sleeve across my eyes.

Some First District cops were forming a line, barking, "Get back! Everybody move back!" I turned around and saw a crowd forming on the sidewalk behind me. There were thirty or forty people already and more coming out of nearby buildings and bars. As I watched, the few dozen people grew to at least a hundred. No wonder. It was late morning in one of the busiest parts of Chicago. We could have a thousand people here soon.

One of the First District cops carried a roll of yellow barrier tape. He tied the end to a light pole and pulled, unrolling it, to the next light pole, where he wrapped tape around and around a few turns, then went on to a third pole.

I heard sirens. Thank heaven—ambulances. The faster they got here, the better. I swiped at my eyes again.

Several cops marched into view from the south side of the building carrying yellow wooden sawhorses. They blocked one lane of State Street on the curb side. A uniformed cop jogged to the center of State Street and with curt jerks of his arm waved curious drivers in idling cars to get moving. Good. The last thing we needed was a gapers' block to slow down the paramedics.

I was still shaking when I saw somebody I knew emerge from the front doors. Hightower is not my favorite Chicago police officer. He is a detective sergeant and very impressed with himself. Slender, a natty dresser, somehow high-stepping, he is a prancing sort of person.

"Sergeant Hightower!"

His gaze swept the crowd. From the way he looked around and then quit looking, it was clear he didn't see anybody important calling him.

"Sergeant Hightower!"

"Oh. Um—Ms. Marsala." He came over to me with no trace of enthusiasm.

"Sergeant Hightower! Can you please get me inside the building?"

"Are you kidding? Of course not!"

"I think the bomb was in McCoo's office!" He was aware I had met McCoo, because of a case a couple of years back. He didn't know we were close friends.

"I don't know whose office it is, but you can't go in." Behind me, an ambulance pulled to the curb, and a paramedic leaped out and raced toward the entrance, carrying a medical case. A second EMT opened the back of the van and unloaded a wheeled stretcher.

Too scared to be cautious, I blurted out, "McCoo is my best friend. I have to see if he's okay!"

"Then you can see from out here."

"Please!"

A second ambulance pulled into a space behind the first one. Hightower said, "Miss Marsala! They've got a very bad situation in there. You know what the elevators are like in this building. Forty years old and slow and small. This is no time to clog them up with an unnecessary person."

"I'll take the stairs."

"Security and Fire are standing by with hoses in the stairwells. Have a little patience. Act like an adult."

At this point the tears overflowed and I had to swipe at my face again. He must have felt some compassion, because he handed me a Kleenex.

"Sergeant Hightower, are there—is it certain that people are injured? Maybe the paramedics are here just to be on the safe side . . ."

He shook his head. He hesitated, then went on, but the crisp, authoritarian tone had left his voice. "No. No, I heard there were injuries. I heard there was at least one fatality."

"No, no."

Please, God, put the clock back.

A second stretcher went in the doors. Hightower and I stared at each other for a moment, almost friends. Then he looked back at the building. Some media types, one with a videocam, were sidling along the CPD wall, looking for an opening to sneak in. Hightower gestured curtly at several uniformed officers, then pointed to the media types, who were now near the doors. The uniforms responded immediately. Hightower wasn't their boss—he was plainclothes and a detective, while they were patrol—but when they saw the problem, they moved fast. The reporters were blocked, reprimanded, and placed squarely outside the barricade.

Three squad cars screamed to a stop on State Street, one in front and two behind the ambulances, augmenting the sawhorses. Their Mars lights flashed, bright even in daylight.

Please, God, put the clock back. All I want is to go back fifteen minutes. That isn't so much to ask, is it? Fifteen minutes. Please, God, put the clock back.

It didn't go back, it went forward slowly. A third ambulance arrived. Several minutes passed agonizingly. Then four uniformed officers erupted from the central door, forming a sort of flying wedge that opened the way for a stretcher. I craned my neck. I'm five feet one, and couldn't see over the people between me and the barrier. "Please! Help me!" I said to Hightower.

The man actually had a heart. "Move over!" he barked at a large woman in a sequined green shirt. "Make a space." He shoved me between the woman and himself.

The stretcher crossed the twenty feet of sidewalk. In a few seconds it would pass out of my sight behind the ambulance. Who was it? I took hold of the barrier tape in one tense hand and squeezed.

I saw dark hair. Maybe McCoo. No, dark *straight* hair. A small face, blood on one cheek. Fred Koy!

He was lying down, an IV running into one arm, but he didn't look dead. They hadn't covered his face.

The ambulance doors slammed behind him. The lights flashed and the siren coughed, then shrieked.

The front doors of the building opened again. As a stretcher emerged, the next ambulance drew forward and shut off my view. I thought, *No, I have to see. If I duck under the tape and run up there, what are they gonna do, shoot me?* But just then the stretcher came around the back of the ambulance into sight. Curly red-blond hair. The patient was in a half-sitting position. She raised her hand, a sooty, dirty hand, and rubbed her eyes. Tracy Shoemaker.

If Hightower was right and someone was dead, the only ones left were McCoo, or Bramble, or Russell Lupinski. It was one of them.

Wait! Couldn't somebody else have walked into the office just after I walked out? Somebody I didn't know could be the fatality.

Lord, what was I doing? Hoping for somebody else to be dead! Somebody I didn't know. It wasn't right to think this way.

But then again, I wasn't hurting anybody. I could hope for whatever I bloody damn well wanted. And what I wanted was my best friend to live.

The doors of the building opened again. At the same moment a fourth ambulance pulled up behind the third. Russell Lupinski lay on the stretcher. Not McCoo. If only it were McCoo. My God, I didn't wish Russell dead; he was the most saturnine of the office staff but he'd always been helpful and nice to me—damn! I couldn't stand this.

Russell was lying down. The left side of his face looked raw and red, as if he had passed under a lawn mower. Why they hadn't covered the wound I couldn't understand. Until the stretcher got closer and I realized that they *had* bandaged him. Blood had soaked through the gauze.

And now the doors opened again. Another stretcher . . .

It was McCoo! It really was! Oh, thank God! Half–sitting up, like Tracy. His big brown face, his wide shoulders—I knew him the second the door opened. Maybe he wasn't badly hurt. He had stayed to be last, of course. He would do that, to make sure everyone else was all right. Like the captain of the ship.

As they trundled the stretcher across the sidewalk, I jumped up and tried to wave encouragement. He didn't see me, or anything else. His eyes were closed. He wasn't dead; he was breathing. In fact, his lips were pulled in, making a bitter, angry line, and his hands were clenched into fists.

No other ambulance arrived. Four. For the five people who worked in McCoo's office.

"But there's a fifth person in that office," I said to Hightower.

"It's a crime scene, Marsala. They won't take the body out for hours."

A crime scene. A body that would lie there for hours, while techs scrabbled over the wreckage and crime-scene photographers made their pictures.

Pictures of Bramble.

◆ 8 ◆

They never let you visit accident victims in hospitals right away unless you're next of kin. They have to examine the patient in the emergency room. They have to "admit the patient." Then a different staff comes in to examine the patient again when he finally gets to his own room. After that the Bomb and Arson Squad was going to be there talking with McCoo. Then, for all I knew, Alcohol, Tobacco and Firearms. The ATF is very big on bombings. Maybe even the FBI. And then, along about 8 P.M., if I was lucky I could probably get in to see him.

I wanted to have something positive for him. Bramble's death would hit him very, very hard.

The top-cops meeting at the CPD no doubt had ended abruptly. "Ended with a bang" crossed my mind, but I was so saddened and numbed by Bramble's death that my brain censored itself almost immediately. Certainly none of the top cops would be holding meetings with reporters today on any subject but the bombing.

Instead of trying to get in the CPD building at Eleventh and State, I went back to the *Chicago Today* offices. There was a possible way to find out who—or at least what sort of person—was leaking to the papers.

I was easily able to catch Barney Ellerway at his desk. He lives at his desk. He has his own one-cup electric tea mug that heats its own water, his own stash of gorp to eat, and, believe it or not, his own small pillow, covered in Black Watch plaid flannel, for catnaps on the desktop. Barney is long on experience, deep of voice, droopy of jowl, and short on hair. What hair he has is sandy, pretty much the same color as his scalp. His eyes are brown, and he wears brown-and-tan tweedy clothing. He looks honest, and he is.

I assumed he'd heard about the bombing, and I started off in the middle of what I wanted to say. "Barney, you've got to tell me something." He blinked. "No, sorry, I take that back. I've got to ask you something."

"Go ahead."

"You've been covering the Shelly Daniello case."

"Yeah. Unpleasant."

"It certainly is. And Barney, you quote 'sources in the department' as giving you inside information."

"Right."

I squirmed. "Um . . . who?"

"You want me to name my inside informant?"

"Barney, I would *never* ask normally. And I would never use him myself, Lord knows, or reveal his name, whoever he is. But you must be aware the target here is Harold McCoo, and I don't believe McCoo's actually trying to hide anything."

"I don't think he would either, usually. But there's something off about the way that shooting is being reported. There's more to it than meets the eye."

"Whatever the Daniello facts are, it's still being used to make McCoo look bad."

"I'll grant you that."

"So who's doing the attacking? Who's giving you this info?"

"I don't know."

"You don't know! Barney, you're the most careful reporter I've ever met. You'd never take a disembodied voice on the phone as giving you gospel."

"Well, this wasn't exactly Deep Throat. About twenty-four hours before the autopsy results were due, I had a call here at the paper asking for me. A voice—whispering—said there were discrepancies between Daniello's story and the facts. He said Daniello had executed her brother-in-law in front of his young daughter. This was Scoopsville, if it was true. 'Cop shoots cop in front of child.' It bleeds and it leads. I asked who my caller was. He wouldn't say. I told him I wouldn't print it if he wouldn't tell me. Then he claimed to have got it from an actual copy of the round table transcript. I said, prove it. The next morning I read the same material in the *Chicago Times*."

"No doubt. They'd print anything."

"So at that point maybe I could have quoted their story. You know the kind of thing: 'Department sources will not confirm or deny the reports in the press that Officer Jurack's four-year-old daughter saw her father gunned down, et cetera, et cetera.' "

"Right."

"But then two days later my guy called back with more information."

"Such as?"

"He said he'd heard that the autopsy discovered a bruise on Jurack's head, proving Daniello had clipped him on the side of the head with her gun, stunning him before she shot him. Which would also mean, given what we know now, that she was closer than she said."

"Uh-oh."

"Uh-oh indeed. Problem was verifying. He still wouldn't tell me who he was. So we were at an impasse, until he said at least he could prove he was an insider."

"Oh, yeah? How?"

"My question exactly. I thought he was gonna say something dumb, like 'I can tell you who the head of Internal Affairs is' or 'I can tell you that Deputy Superintendent Bannister never misses a chance to make disparaging remarks about Spurlark. Calls Spurlark the honky turkey.' Which he does, and it's actually pretty funny, because of the way Spurlark walks around kind of gobbling at people. Anyway, dumb stuff that everybody knows or could find out just by asking around."

"But?"

"But he blew me away by saying he could tell me everything that went on at the superintendent's meeting last week. The only people regularly at the weekly meeting are the superintendent himself, the four deputy superintendents, an ADS to take notes, and the CPD lawyer. Once in a while they have the head of the FOP, or the district commanders, or whatever, but not always, and I knew they hadn't last week."

"He could be bluffing."

"Yes, except I have an—ah—contact who could verify it. In fact, I asked him to quote me some stuff and I did take it to my guy. It checked out, right down to the remark by Winter that if the deli didn't send up some kind of doughnut other than jelly, he was going to start bringing his own. Apparently he got grape jelly on his shirt. Winter is particular about his clothes."

"So you have an insider, an *insider's* insider—"

"Don't get fixated on that. To continue. Whoever my Deep Throat is, he'd been there. At the meeting. Unless he bugged the superintendent's office. That's a joke. They sweep that office immediately before every meeting. I thought maybe he got somebody to tell him what went on. If he had, he would have prepared some tasty tidbits for me, but he wouldn't have memorized the entire contents of the meeting. So I asked him a couple of specific questions, ordinary budget stuff. He gave me answers. Then I checked his answers with my guy. He was right on both."

"That's convincing."

"Damn right. Then he got me a copy of a page of the report from the medical examiner. And I printed the story. Whatever else he is, Deep Throat's certainly an informed source."

"Deep Throat is a top cop."

"I think so."

"How do you know Deep Throat isn't your regular contact?"

"I couldn't tell from the voice because he whispered. But my guy wouldn't need . . . hmmm. I see what you mean. If he wanted to tell me something more sensitive than usual, and didn't want me to know where it came from—"

"Or if he didn't want you to realize he was specifically trying to damage Harold McCoo."

"That's possible. McCoo is tremendously popular."

I said, "Yes, or if he was planning to send this bomb today to blow up McCoo if nothing else worked."

"What! What bomb?"

"You haven't heard?"

"I've heard nothing. I've been at my desk all morning."

So I told him. He was stunned, saddened, and outraged, in that order. But at the same time I could sense his mental wheels going around, trying to put this together with the rest of his story, trying to see how it fit. After a few seconds, another thought crossed his mind.

"Jeez, Cat. I hope nothing I wrote gave the bomber the idea."

"How?"

"Made somebody mad at McCoo."

"Somebody was already mad at McCoo."

"I mean, like Jurack's family."

"You can't pull your punches writing just because you may set off some nut. Plus I don't think Jurack's family would have the inside knowledge to send this bomb this way. It has to have been a letter bomb, maybe in a court-tape cassette. I've seen them in Bramble's in-box when I walk by her desk. I am more upset than anybody that the press has been helping sling mud at McCoo. But the press isn't causing this. The attack's coming from a person who stands to gain an advantage."

"I know. I know."

"And it could be your friend in high places."

"If he's done anything that wrong, he's not my friend."

*   *   *

Eight P.M. I walked along the hospital corridor looking for McCoo's room, feeling some trepidation. He'd been depressed enough by the personal attacks. Bramble and I, or maybe his own common sense, had managed to cheer him up. But the murder of Bramble, his aide and confidante for so many years, would be a crushing blow.

Outside the closed door of one of the private rooms was a chair and a seated uniformed cop. This must be McCoo's room.

"I need to see Harold McCoo," I said.

"*Chief* Harold McCoo."

"That's the one."

"You can't go in there."

"Hey, I know you need to guard him. I know you don't want another bombing. But I'm a friend. Just tell him Cat Marsala is outside and see what he says."

The man looked skeptical, and his eyes scanned my body to see if I was carrying any obvious weapons—explosives, guns, machetes. Male officers are not allowed to body-search females, of course, and I was afraid he would just send me away, claiming there was no woman officer to make a search. However, male officers are allowed to run their baton over women, and with the tip of a baton you can easily feel metal objects like knives and guns. I was about to suggest he try this when he suddenly got up and went into McCoo's room, carefully closing the door behind himself. I was glad they were taking care of McCoo. As far as I was concerned, the guard could do anything he wanted to ensure that I was harmless. He'd get no complaints from me. He could even pat me down if he wanted to.

But he came back and said, "Okay. You can go in."

McCoo was seated upright against the bed back like a mahogany Buddha. There was a bandage over half of his skull on the right side. That was all. Maybe that meant his injuries weren't too bad. I stopped just three steps inside the door, expecting depression.

I saw fury.

"They *killed* Bramble, Cat," he said, so softly that I knew he was even more angry than he looked. I walked toward the bed. As I watched, he squeezed a plastic cup of reddish stuff that looked like cranberry juice. The cup deformed, then cracked, and the juice ran all over his sleeve. Muttering, "You and I are spilling a lot of beverages these days," I threw tissues from a box beside his bed onto his arm and the sheet, but he hardly noticed and went on talking. He didn't really even look at me, but he talked. The depressed McCoo, a stranger to me, was gone. I hadn't often seen McCoo angry, and never this angry, but at least this was the man I knew and liked.

"Bramble was an utterly good person," he said. "She wasn't necessarily a *comfortable* person, but she was a good person."

"Did she have family?"

"A mother. A grown son, born when she was a teenager."

"I see. McCoo, I'm embarrassed to ask this. I never knew her name."

"Her name? Serafina. Serafina Barnes Bramble."

McCoo looked away for a few seconds. I waited. I threw the soaked tissues into the ugly aqua plastic wastebasket and patted some more Kleenex on the stains on the sheet and McCoo's wrist.

"You are going on with what we talked about," McCoo said, not asking a question.

"Yes, I went to see a reporter I know. He says basically that you were right. The leaks are from inside the department."

"That was already obvious. How high up?"

"Top cops."

McCoo said, "I knew it. Can you get him to tell you who?"

"No. He doesn't know. He verified the contents of the leaks through a contact of his, but it's a Deep Throat kind of situation."

"Hell."

"When will you be back in your office?"

"Tomorrow. The office will be livable. There was a small fire but I got the fire extinguisher on it and then Security finished the job. Some of the papers on Bramble's desk were burned and so were a very few papers left out around the main office that caught fire when pieces of burning stuff flew around. We're supposed to be back in tomorrow."

A voice in the doorway said, "But *you* won't."

The voice came from a small black woman wearing a powder-blue-and-white-striped dress and a blue scarf tied over her hair like a turban. She was chubby without being fat, dumpling-like, with rounded hips and bosom, and a nipped-in small waist. Her face was rounded, and a few laugh lines showed that it was ordinarily used for smiling. She was very angry.

"You're staying here the full forty-eight hours!" she said.

"Um, Cat. This is my wife, Susanne."

I said, "I'm happy to have a chance to meet you."

She said, "Good afternoon." But her tone of voice implied not that she was happy to meet me, too, but that she'd be happy to chew me up and spit me out.

McCoo had talked a lot about Susanne over the years. She had had breast cancer a year ago, which frightened him badly, though he had expressed his fear as anger. She'd had surgery and chemo and was supposedly all right. Probably she wore the turban-style scarf because she liked it, not because she had lost hair.

"Susanne, don't look daggers at Cat," McCoo said. "She's going to help me out."

"You don't need help, you need rest. What you *really* don't need right now is talking business. If she wants to help so much, she can leave."

"Susanne!"

I said, "Listen, I know he's been injured. I just had a message for him, but I'll go now."

Susanne relented a little. "He's got a very bad concussion. They're keeping him another day."

McCoo said, "Oh, no, they're not."

"Oh, yes, they are."

"Oh, no, they're not."

I said, "I saw him when the paramedics were taking him out, and I thought since he was sitting up and looking alert, he was okay—"

"When they got him here, he couldn't remember anything that happened before the explosion," Susanne said, "and the neurologist said the nausea he's having isn't a good sign, either. So they're keeping him."

"Well, I remember it perfectly now," McCoo said. "ATF thinks it was a letter bomb, Cat."

"That was pretty obvious. You get all those fat envelopes."

"Somebody sent it to me in the mail. But Bramble opens my mail—opened my mail. Bramble never let the mail sit around more than two minutes—"

"So why were you injured?" I said hastily, trying to get his mind off Bramble. "There's a wall between you and the outer office."

"I wasn't in my office. I went into the outer office to ask Bramble for a formset. But then Tracy asked me to look at something, and I went over to her desk. And right then the bomb blew."

"If you'd been closer to Bramble, you'd have been killed," Susanne said, the pitch of her voice rising. "We . . . I wouldn't be here right now. You'd be dead and I'd be at the funeral parlor picking out a casket—oh, God! And now you have the nerve not to take the doctor's advice!"

"Well, I'm *not* dead," McCoo said.

"This is like old times," I said. "I remember once when I was hurt in an explosion, and you came to the hospital to see me. If I remember correctly, you came to find out some details about the explosion and who was where, and when I said I wanted to leave, you told me not to until I was discharged and to be nice to the doctors. And do what they told me to."

"Did he really?" Susanne said meaningfully.

"He did. He surely did." This was not totally accurate, but close enough.

She said, "Thanks."

❖ 9 ❖

When I entered the chief of detectives' office the next morning, the first thing I noticed was that the ancient linoleum floor was blackened over an amoeba-shaped area near the wall. There was an unburned, square area where the side of Bramble's desk had stood. The desk itself had blocked the flames from reaching that part of the wall. Just above, a flare of soot flowed up the wall like a dusky flower blossom.

The desk was gone, her chair was gone, her bookcase was gone, and she was gone.

There were no guards. Probably there was nothing left to guard.

The room was dark, as if still tinged with the soot and smoke of the explosion. The air smelled of carbon and ashes. But the darkness was not caused by lingering smoke or by the miasma of sadness and horror. Two of the fluorescent fixtures, the middle ones directly over Bramble's desk, were missing, wires hanging raw from the conduits, and there were plywood boards over three of the windows, all but the farthest-back window near Fred Koy's desk. As if on a whim, the bomb had left his window miraculously intact, scarcely even cracked. Fresh tubes glowed in the overhead fluorescent fixtures at the front and back ends of the ceiling, but the fixtures themselves were smoky. Except for Tracy's desk, every surface in the entire room was grayed with soot.

In the front of the room the bracket that had held the fire extinguisher was empty. McCoo had put out the fire with it. There was still one extinguisher near the hall door—the old halon type that was no longer sold, I think because halon damages the ozone layer. McCoo had been lucky his still worked.

A bunch of yellow barrier tape lay wadded into a ball in the wastebasket nearest me. Obviously the main office had been released for use, but McCoo's door stood ajar and there were sounds of strange men talking in his office.

From his desk at the back of the room, Fred Koy noticed me and waved. "Cat!" he said. "I hear you saw the boss."

"Yes, and he was under heavy guard, you might say. Both a cop and Susanne."

Koy and I averted our eyes from the blackened wall where Bramble had worked and in fact had lived for many years. Tracy Shoemaker entered from the hall at this moment, carrying a pail and several rags. The sleeves of her blue uniform blouse were rolled up. Tracy was a medium-sized woman, maybe five feet five, with freckles on her nose and reddish-blond hair. "I'm cleaning," she said, scarcely glancing at us. "The janitors didn't do a thing." She immediately dipped a rag and wrung it out until it was damp but not dripping and began swabbing the windowsill near her desk. The desk itself was already the cleanest in the room. She scrubbed the sill with enough energy to bunch the muscles in her forearm.

People deal with shock in many ways.

"How are you both?" I asked.

"Scalp cut," Koy said cheerfully. "Bled a lot. Didn't add up to much."

"Shouldn't you both take the day off?"

"And leave the boss with this mess?"

There was a three-inch railroad track of stitches down his scalp, from the crown of his head to right above the ear. The cut was a lot bigger than he implied. Tracy's hair had been trimmed since yesterday, and I deduced that some of it had been burned, and the rest had been evened up to match. "I was just knocked out," she said. "I guess I was lucky."

"Letter bombs aren't usually very powerful," Koy said. "I

took a class on them a few years ago. They're"—he hesitated
a second—"selective. Surgical."

I said, "It was small? Small enough so that it might not
have . . . killed anybody?"

Koy said, "Sure, maybe. Remember that several ones the
Unabomber sent didn't kill the target."

We were talking as if it were a case, the bomb a device for
detectives and techs to deal with, not a deadly weapon that
had murdered a friend. And it was probably good that we
were.

"They're small, yes," Koy went on, "but they're very
focused. You take some C-4 and put it in a videotape cassette,
for instance. Real commonplace method. You put backing on
one side and put the detonator in the other side. The detonator is just like a blasting cap, or like the 'solar igniters' that
kids use to fire model rockets. In fact, you can even use a detonator from a car air bag for a trigger. Where you put the detonator determines which side of the C-4 blows out."

"Yes, but it must have been in a mailing envelope. You
wouldn't be able to know which side the vic—uh—the person
who opened it was going to be facing."

"Sure you would. You put it in a padded envelope, the kind
that has a pull tab to open. People always face the tab when
they pull it. Same with a FedEx envelope. They face the pull
tab. Think how awkward it would be the other way around."

"I guess that's right. You think the bomb was in a tape case?
It seemed likely to me."

"The techs found fragments of the outside of a video cassette."

"With any evidence of who sent it? Was any of the envelope left? Was there a return address? Wouldn't Bramble have
been suspicious of an envelope without a return address?"

"It probably did have one. Why not? How hard is that to
fake? Anyhow, with us getting so many court videotapes,
who'd ever think it was unusual?"

Tracy threw her rag in the bucket with a splash. "I don't

want to talk about this!" she said. "I want you both to stop talking about this, right *now!*"

"Sure thing, Trace," Koy said.

Fred's manner was perfectly healthy, I thought, even if it annoyed Tracy. Fred, who was always cheerful anyhow, was experiencing the ebullience of survival, the sheer thrill of having been close to death and cheating it. To a certain extent he was also trying to make sense of what had happened. Tracy's attempt to avoid thinking about it and to wash away all the physical traces was not going to help her in the long run.

"McCoo will probably be back tomorrow," I said. "They were just keeping him for observation."

"Observation of what?" Fred asked.

"Yeah, they wouldn't keep him if there wasn't something wrong," Tracy said.

"Apparently he had a very severe concussion."

Fred said, "Oh."

"Lupinski not back yet either?" I asked.

"No. We heard he had to have surgery on his ear."

"Oh. That's a shame." I pointed at McCoo's office. "Who's in there?"

"Bomb and Arson, I guess," Fred said. "And some techie guys. Maybe ATF techies."

I wandered over and peered into McCoo's inner office. There was comparatively little soot and no damage whatever to his window. I guess the bomb really was as surgical as Fred said. It killed the person who opened the envelope and nobody else. Three men were sorting through papers. They gave me a brief glance, but since I didn't enter, they went back to work. I noticed that the glass carafe of McCoo's coffee-maker was cracked. "We can't have that," I said.

Tracy said, "What?"

"McCoo without a coffeemaker."

"Don't you people realize what's happened?" Tracy shouted. "Bramble's been *murdered.* She's dead, and she's never coming back! She's dead *forever!*"

Lord.

"I know that, Tracy." I put my arm around her shoulders. "I miss her. But I can't do anything about it. I can't make things right."

Tracy spun away and started furiously washing the wall near where Bramble's desk had been.

It occurred to me that Tracy could benefit a little by actually helping—by doing something real, not just erasing soot. And she was usually the office audio person.

"Tracy, do you have a copy of the tape of the radio traffic during the Ben Jurack shooting?"

"Of course." She paused with a wet rag in one hand and the other hand balled into a fist and propped on her hip.

"Could I listen to it?"

"I guess. The boss said to help you." Reluctantly, she hung her rag over the pail.

Tapes were filed in a specially constructed cabinet with tape-sized shelves that rolled in and out. Tracy searched for the one with the correct date and time, got out a player, plugged it in, inserted the tape, fast-forwarded a few seconds, and said, "There."

She stepped away to her desk as if rejecting the whole event. Still, I noticed she did not resume her washing, but stood and listened.

"Chicago Police Department point-to-point radio; fifteen-thirty hours."

"Eighteen thirty-one. One-eight-three-one." This meant the dispatcher was calling car 1831—Eighteenth District, car thirty-one.

The patrol car answered, *"Eighteen thirty-one."*

"We've got a bus alarm, city number 322, westbound on Division."

"Any idea what's the problem?"

"No, but school's just let out."

"*Oh. Right you are. Kids! Ten-four, squad.*"

"*Eighteen thirty-three, can you take a number-two parker at—hang on a minute. Let me change that. Can you handle— you a ten-four unit today, thirty-three?*"

"*Ten-four, squad.*" This meant he was a two-man unit. If it had been a one-man unit, he would have responded, "Ten ninety-nine."

"*Possible drive-by shooting at Hollis East High School. Victim's supposed to be in the basketball court. Outdoor basketball court. Fire's responding.*" "Fire" meant a fire-department ambulance.

"*Ten-four.*"

"*Eighteen thirty-seven. One-eight-three-seven.*"

"*Three-seven. I suppose you're going to give us your number-two parker.*" It was a woman's voice. It must be Shelly Daniello.

"*I wish. No, I'm going to send you a little bit out of your sector, but thirty-three's tied up. Got a domestic violence. Neighbor called it in. Seventeen sixty-four Barcourt on the one.*" By "on the one" they mean first floor.

"*Uh, sure, squad. Any name on that?*" She seemed to be hoping it was some other apartment than her sister's. I could hear the tension in her voice. Probably I wouldn't have noticed if I hadn't known the background and been primed to listen.

"*Jurack. Jurack is the name.*"

With maybe some hope remaining, she asked, "*Jurack is the complainant, or—*"

"*Nope. Complainant is citizen. Mr. Citizen.*"

"*Ten-four, squad. We're coming from Superior and Lake Shore.*"

"*Well, make it as fast as you can. Caller said there's a lot of screaming.*"

So there it was. I wondered whether the talk of screaming had strung her nerves up tighter, and had made the shooting more likely.

I waited for five or six minutes, listening for car 1837 or Officer Daniello's voice, while sounds of the other radio traffic went past me. The drive-by shooting at the school unraveled tragically. A child had been shot. The ambulance arrived. Within three minutes the beat car had located four teenaged kids in a deteriorated Ford Bronco, arrested them, and found guns in the car.

Finally I heard, "*Eighteen thirty-seven. I have an emergency!*" It was a man's voice.

If he had been calling about an officer in danger, he would have said, "Ten-one." So the dispatcher knew, as I did, that it was some other sort of emergency.

"*All units stay off the air. Eighteen thirty-seven has an emergency. Go ahead, thirty-seven.*"

"*I need an ambulance at this location.*"

"*Ten-four, thirty-seven.*"

"*I have an injured civilian. I also need a supervisor at this location.*" In the background, I could hear screaming. I couldn't tell whether a woman or a child was screaming. Unless it was a man shrieking, high-pitched, in pain.

"*I have Fire responding to seventeen sixty-four Barcourt on the one. Right, thirty-seven?*"

"*Ten-four, squad.*" There was tension in the man's voice. In the background a woman's voice, barely audible, said, "*Keep back.*" Somebody, somewhere, was sobbing.

One of my questions was answered for sure. This was not a setup. Nobody had arranged to get Officer Shelly Daniello sent to the home of her own sister. Daniello's squad car had not even been on that beat that day. With a possible drive-by shooting tying up the regular beat car, the dispatcher had to pick the next nearest car, even though it covered a different sector. Shelly Daniello's disaster had come upon her by sheer chance.

The bombing was the lead story in all the headlines. News anchors on the local morning shows spoke breathlessly that "crime came to the very heart of Chicago's crime-fighting establishment yesterday, when a bomb exploded on the eighth floor of the Chicago Police Department, killing one and injuring four." Superintendent Spurlark appeared from a variety of angles on the morning news shows. On "Channel Two News" he was seen in a dramatic low-angle shot, saying, "The Bomb and Arson squad has recovered significant evidence and we hope to have a lead to the bomber shortly." Cut to Spurlark in a more distant shot, showing a forest of reporters: "My people are on the job. We're actively following leads at this moment." Then he turned from the reporters with a waving-away motion of his hand that meant, "I'm so busy," and strode away. Knowing Spurlark, he strode briskly to his office, where he spent twenty active minutes yelling at his ADS.

The likelihood of one of the top cops' being willing to talk with a reporter today was somewhere between zero and none. They would be very guarded, which wouldn't help me at all. Let the dust settle. I could talk with them tomorrow.

I phoned McCoo at the hospital.

"You told me you knew Shelly Daniello, right?"

"Cat, you wouldn't believe the coffee in this place. They're trying to kill me."

"Focus, McCoo. Do you know Daniello personally?"

"They're trying to *make* me walk out."

"Don't. Susanne would be furious. Now, I know you're irritated, but just answer my question. Do you know Shelly Daniello personally?"

"I don't know what 'personally' means. People keep saying they know the mayor 'personally.' Can you know somebody impersonally? Okay, okay, don't snarl at me. After the ice-ball case that I told you about, she came and thanked me."

"So she likes you? Trusts you?"

"Probably."

"Can you give her a call and ask her to meet with me?"

Cops need to hear from other cops that you're okay before they'll talk with you. Especially if you're a reporter, and most especially when the case is as sensitive as this one.

Daniello lived in a second-floor apartment in Old Town. Well, the edge of Old Town, actually, walking distance from the El and walking distance from the good restaurants in the area, but outside the high-rent district. Her apartment was even smaller than mine: if a burner on the kitchen gas stove was on, she'd be taking a risk of explosion by spraying her hair in the bathroom.

In that small a space you either have to be compulsively neat or otherwise give up and throw everything everywhere. She was the neat type. She had very few possessions—one easy chair, one hard chair near a small desk, no sofa. A single bed in an alcove. Shelly Daniello definitely was not set up for house guests. Or for gentlemen callers, either, I thought.

She was tall, very slender, with long arms and legs and a lot of chestnut hair that had more red than brown in it. She reminded me of a racehorse—a racehorse *before* the race. She kept an eye on me as she let me in, almost as if I were a gatekeeper and she might have to bolt from the starting gate at any moment. She paced in a circle while she talked. She said, "Look, I don't know how I can help McCoo, and I don't know if he can help me, either." She practically pawed the floor. I knew what was wrong. She was a cop; she was on suspension; she was bored and wanted to get back on the job.

"A person like you must have a real problem in this small a space," I said.

She reared back and stared.

I said, "I have a small apartment too, but I don't have as much extra physical energy as you do."

Shelly Daniello decided not to be insulted. "Okay," she said. Reluctantly, she added, "Let's sit, then." She actually smiled at me, but I noticed she took the hard chair and left me the soft one. No wonder this woman didn't own a sofa. She wouldn't know what to do with it.

She said, "If McCoo says you can help, I have to at least believe he means it. That's one very straight guy."

"Yeah, he is."

"But I still think it's hopeless. I think they're out to get me. See, there's a lot of shit involved here that the department wants to cover up. There are more cops who beat their wives and children than the department wants to admit."

I nodded. "There are a lot of abusers in the general population, too."

"Yes, but cops can be authoritarian. Some of them go into that line of work because they like to push people around. Anyhow, the CPD left Jurack on the job. A guy who had several abuse calls to his home plus a lot of excessive force complaints on the job. That can't look good for them."

"Tell me what happened at the Jurack house."

She jumped back up, swung around and stared at the ceiling, changing gears mentally. Turning to face me, she said in a clear, unemotional voice, "It was fifteen thirty-one hours. My partner and I were on patrol in a sector just north of the Loop. I thought we were about to be given a different call, some sort of parking violation, as I remember, when the dispatcher gave us the 1764 Barcourt address. I knew it was my sister's address, but we're supposed to respond anyway."

"I know."

"We responded immediately. They're northwest of where we were, and it only took us six or seven minutes tops to get there. I entered the premises and discovered Jurack in the act of attacking my sister with a knife. I cautioned him, but he lunged at us, and fearing for her life and mine, I fired at him. He was struck in the chest. My partner called for an ambulance. Jurack died at the scene, even though they didn't pronounce him until he got to the hospital."

"Officer Daniello, that's okay as far as it goes, but I've already read the report. I don't want police lingo. I want to know what *happened*. What you felt. What you saw. What you heard. What you smelled. Would you tell it to me in full detail, and without the police jargon? Please?"

She studied me coolly for a few seconds. I could almost see her making a decision, then acting on it. There was no agonizing for the benefit of the observer. She placed her feet about shoulder-width apart, clasped her hands behind her back, and simply began again.

"It was just about three-thirty, a bright, sunny day. You know how crystal-clear March can be. Schools were letting out. It was a Friday, which means more—um—*vigor* on the part of the school kids. There was a drive-by shooting in our district, which tied up one or two cars. When we got the call, Brad, my partner, was annoyed. He always hated domestic-violence calls, talked about how we weren't 'baby-sitters' and how people ought to straighten out their own lives.

"I didn't let on at first that it might be my sister's address or that her husband was a cop, because all Brad would have done is bitch and moan even worse the whole way there. But when we got within three minutes or so of the building, I said, 'The asshole we're gonna arrest is my brother-in-law.'

"Brad didn't like that much, either, but he knew the rules as well as I did, and we jumped out of the car and went racing into the house. Brad was wearing his damned sunglasses, which he thinks make him look just as slick as hot shit on ice, and he must've bumped into the wall where the hall makes a turn. Practically knocked himself out, but I didn't know that at the time.

"I knew the house well, of course, and I could hear screaming from the back, and I knew they were in a room they call the 'television room.' It isn't a big apartment. All the rooms are little, but there's this one off the other side of the kitchen, the side away from the dining room, where they have their television set and a sofa and a recliner, and they keep the shades down a little because it's just for television. So being near the kitchen and all, I guessed right away that the fight had started in there, and I realized later that was why Jurack had a knife."

"You're saying the knife was unusual?"

"Yes. Usually he basically just hit her. He stabbed her with scissors once, maybe four years ago, just before Beanbag—Belinda—was born. We nicknamed her Beanbag because she got nuts about playing beanbag when she was about two. That kid could play beanbag all day long, no joke. Well. Anyway." A look of distress crossed her face when she mentioned Belinda. I assumed she was the child who had been in the house when Daniello shot Jurack.

"Go on."

"Usually he just beat her—my sister, I mean—with fists. The last time the police were called—I wasn't on duty at the time and I went to the hospital later to see her—he had whipped her with the cord from the electric clock. You could actually see the imprint of the plug, like a wedge shape with two prongs, on her back and thighs. In a few places the plug's prongs had hit and you could see these two holes like she'd been bitten by a giant snake. Well, anyway.

"I ran through the kitchen toward the screams and when I got to the door of the room, Jurack was silhouetted against the window and he was raising his arm up. I saw the knife and a gleam off the blade. I yelled, 'Freeze! Police!' instead of saying who I was, because he didn't have any respect for me, either, any more than he did for her. But he knew my voice

right away, and he just laughed. He said, 'Hey! It's the cop-
bitch. A whole family of bitches!'

"My sister was screaming, 'He'll cut you! He'll cut you!'
but she didn't do anything except scream, hadn't even called
the cops. She backed up toward me, though. Jurack said, 'Two
for the price of one! I been wishing for this!' and he sort of
stalked one step toward me. I had my side arm out by then
and I said, 'One step more and I shoot.' He just laughed. He
said something about—well, he said something like 'You're
too pussy to shoot' and he stalked, not walked but really
stalked, a couple of steps toward my sister and me. Then he
slashed out toward me. And I fired."

"Was he close enough to touch you when he slashed out?"

"Not quite. But he was close enough to my sister."

I waited but she didn't go on, so I said, "Did he fall?"

"No, he slashed out again first, and then he fell. My sister was
bleeding, and my partner was standing someplace behind
me—he'd just come in the door. Don't know whether he'd
been hanging outside because he was scared, or what. I heard
him key his radio, calling for an ambulance. I went to check
Jurack, but I looked for the knife first, because for all I knew he
was faking. The knife was on the floor in front of him and he was
coughing up blood. He was on his stomach, but his face was
turned enough for me to see. And just then Beanbag must've
come in, because she kind of toddled over toward her dad and
I looked at her and she said"—Daniello choked a little now—
"she came over to Jurack and she said, 'Daddy?' "

I let the words hang for several seconds more, hoping she
might add something else, something about how she felt, but
she didn't. She kept a poker face all the while. It was only in
her tone of voice that I could read her emotions.

"So Jurack lay with the knife in front of him—"

"He was near the sofa. He was still alive, but sluggish. You
know how it is with serious injuries? Sometimes they don't
realize how bad they're hurt at first. They're talking and
everything, like it was a normal day. And then the shock and

blood loss kick in, and they start to go on you. Jurack had that
sleepy note in his voice. The kind that makes you say, this guy
isn't going to last more than a few minutes."

"What did your sister do?"

"Not a hell of a lot. While I was trying to stop Belinda from
walking into the blood, saying, 'Keep back' and stuff, Marie
was standing over Jurack, too, but it was weird. She hated
him, partly, and thought she loved him, partly, and while she
stood there, you could see her kind of tremble back and forth.
It was like a science-fiction movie where the person has been
taken over by a spirit and their hand wants to kill but their
mind says no and they're kind of fighting themselves, one
hand like holding the other back?"

"I can imagine."

"She bent over him and just jittered back and forth. I had
to tell her, 'Take care of Belinda. Get her out of here.' Belinda
needed to be gotten away from her father. She was just standing there, staring with these big, liquid eyes, me with one
hand on her shoulder. I was trying to give Marie something to
do, too, telling her to get the kid away. But I shouldn't have
had to tell her. You'd think she'd've known enough—"

"Shock does funny things to people."

"Especially when it's a life of shocks."

There wasn't much I could say to that.

"I was going to elevate his feet and all, but then I thought,
Save the scene for the detectives if he dies. There was nothing you could put a tourniquet on. He was hit in the chest,
dead-center. That's a pun, isn't it? Dead-center?"

"Sort of."

"When Marie led Beanbag out, the kid had her hands—
see, Beanbag was wearing these bib overalls that she just
loved. She said they made her look 'like the music videos.'
She saw them on television. And she was hunched over and
had her hands buried behind the bib part of the bib overalls,
so Marie couldn't take her hand. She had to kind of put her
palm on the back of Beanbag's neck and steer her away."

"All right. You're sure the child wasn't there when you ran into the room."

"Yes, I'm sure."

"How? How can you be positive?"

"Look, I'm a cop. We're trained to be observant. You enter some kind of crisis situation, somebody might have a gun, somebody might be behind the door or whatever, you learn to look. Your life depends on it."

"But this was an apartment you were familiar with, and an attacker you knew all about."

"True . . ."

"So you wouldn't have been looking out for a second assailant behind the door."

"That's true." She paused in midstride and did me the compliment of seriously considering what I had said. Her eyes moved as if she was mentally replaying the incident. "Yes, that's true. All I can tell you," she said after four or five seconds, "is this. I think I do it habitually. I think I scan all the rooms I go into. I do it on duty and off duty. I do it in restaurants. I do it in movie theaters. By now, I don't think I can help it."

"I'll buy that. My second question, Officer Daniello. How far were you from Jurack when you fired?"

"Three or four feet. When he stalked toward me, it was just two steps. He was holding his knife out and it never touched me. No matter who asks, or how many times they ask. It's still three or four feet."

"Pardon me, but how do you know?"

"How does anybody know anything? I can picture it. Did you drive here? How do you know where you parked your car?"

"I remember driving up and finding a spot near the corner. I understand what you're saying. It's just that in the Jurack situation it all must have happened so fast."

"It's like a snapshot. He's coming at me—actually toward me and my sister both—and the knife is out in front of him. I think he's going for her, but he keeps coming directly at me. And I fire."

"All right. One last thing: I'm sure you've heard that Jurack had some blunt trauma to the side of his head—"

"I sure have heard about it. It's part of the reason I'm suspended. I don't know how it got there."

"You didn't hit him?"

"I didn't hit him. Never. Except with a lead slug, of course, if you count that."

"I'm not trying to trap you. I just need to be sure."

"Well, I didn't hit him. Maybe Marie hit him earlier during the fight, before I got there. I sure hope she did. Bet she didn't, though. As far as I know, she never fought back. She was so scared of him."

"Too bad."

"Don't you believe me? You know, I'm getting damn tired of not being believed."

"I don't *dis*believe you. For McCoo's sake I need to get a clear picture—"

"You're doing just what they all do."

"What?"

"Trying to catch me in some contradiction. Find something that doesn't square with some of the other evidence. Let me explain police work to you, Ms. Marsala. In the real world, in every investigation, there are odds and ends left over. 'Clues' that don't fit anywhere. Two perfectly honest people who saw one scene and remember it two utterly different ways. The footprint of somebody you can never locate. Whatever. That's the real world. A police round table ought to realize that."

"Didn't the FOP attorney tell you to stop and think it over before you gave them all the details—I mean—"

"I waived my right to an attorney."

"Why?"

"Look, I don't think you understand the sequence of events here. I shot Jurack in self-defense, and defending my sister.

WAIVER OF COUNSEL/REQUEST TO SECURE COUNSEL
CHICAGO POLICE DEPARTMENT

NAME OF ACCUSED	RANK	STAR NO	UNIT OF ASSIGNMENT
Shelly M. Daniello	p	31293	18

☐ **WAIVER OF COUNSEL**

I, the undersigned, hereby acknowledge that I have received and read the charges/allegations against me and I knowingly and voluntarily wish to proceed with the hearing, examination or interrogation without having counsel of my own choosing present to advise me during this hearing, examination or interrogation.

Date-Time ___3/7/97___   Signature ___Shelly M Daniello___

☐ **REQUEST TO SECURE LEGAL COUNSEL**

I, the undersigned, having been advised of my right to counsel of my own choosing at all hearings, examinations and interrogations in connection with the charges/allegations against me which have been given to me in writing and receipt of which is hereby acknowledged, elect to secure the services of counsel and agree to proceed with said hearing, examination or interrogation at

_____ hours, on _____, 19_____, in Room _____

_____ Chicago, Illinois, at which time said hearing, examination or interrogation shall be commenced. By placing my signature upon this statement, I affirm my wish to secure said counsel and agree to comply with Department hearing, examination or interrogation scheduled on the date aforesaid.

Date-Time _____   Signature _____

WITNESSES _____

DISTRIBUTION
COMPLAINT REGISTER INVESTIGATION

Original to investigator's file
Duplicate to affected member

COMPLAINT REGISTER NO ___D7783___
                        c-0
ATTACHMENT NO ___2___

CPD-44 106 (Rev 10/93)

As far as I knew at the time, my partner was right behind me and saw me fire in self-defense. Simple. No problem."

"Well, but a round table is an inquiry. Like a trial."

"Wait a minute! A round table is routine. In Chicago, *every time* a police officer fires his gun on duty, a round table is held immediately. Even if you're a sniper and took out a guy who was about to blow the head off the President of the United States. Even if you're in the locker room getting dressed and your gun discharges by accident."

"All right. I understand. It's routine."

"Here. Here's the waiver."

She went to a drawer in the side table and got out some papers. Flipping through, she found one and shoved it at me.

"See? So I go to the round table and waive an attorney, thinking, No problem. The second thing you need to know is that a cop has to answer questions put to him or her by a superior officer. You have no right to remain silent."

"What? What about the Constitution?"

"Here."

She shoved another sheet at me. It was headed "Administrative Proceedings Rights."

"Look at number four," she said. " 'You have no right to remain silent.' "

"But this is wrong! This is unconstitutional!"

"Well, see, you have the idea that a police department is a democracy. It's more like an army. A cop *can* refuse to answer, and a cop has constitutional rights, but if I don't answer the legitimate questions of a superior officer, I can be fired. Look down at number six: 'Your discharge will be sought.' "

"What they're saying is if you exercise your constitutional right not to incriminate yourself, you can be fired."

"In a nutshell."

"Jeez."

"It's no secret. All police departments work this way, as far as I know."

ADMINISTRATIVE PROCEEDINGS RIGHTS (Statutory) CHICAGO POLICE DEPARTMENT			GIVEN TO MEMBER DATE		TIME
NAME OF ACCUSED SHELLY M. DANIELLO	RANK P	STAR NO 31293	UNIT OF ASSIGNMENT 18		

The law provides that you are to be advised of the following:

1. Any admission or statement made by you in the course of this hearing, interrogation or examination may be used as the basis for your suspension or as the basis for charges seeking your removal or discharge or suspension in excess of 30 days.

2. You have the right to counsel of your choosing to be present with you to advise you at this hearing, interrogation or examination and you may consult with him as you desire.

3. You have a right to be given a reasonable time to obtain counsel of your own choosing.

4. You have no right to remain silent. You have an obligation to truthfully answer questions put to you. You are advised that your statements or responses constitute an official police report.

5. If you refuse to answer questions put to you, you will be ordered by a superior officer to answer the questions.

6. If you persist in your refusal after the order has been given to you, you are advised that such refusal constitutes a violation of the Rules and Regulations of the Chicago Police Department and will serve as a basis for which your discharge will be sought.

7. You are further advised that by law any admission or statement made by you during the course of this hearing, interrogation or examination and the fruits thereof cannot be used against you in a subsequent criminal proceeding.

_____

The undersigned hereby acknowledges that he was informed of the above rights.

Signature *Shelly M Daniello*

WITNESSES *Albert Kannamanye* DC

_____

DISTRIBUTION
COMPLAINT REGISTER INVESTIGATION

Original to investigator's file
Duplicate to affected member

CPD-44 105 (Rev 10/93)

COMPLAINT REGISTER NO D7783

ATTACHMENT NO 4

CRIMINAL RIGHTS
CHICAGO POLICE DEPARTMENT

GIVEN TO ACCUSED
DATE   TIME

NAME OF ACCUSED	RANK	STAR NO.	UNIT OF ASSIGNMENT

You are hereby advised that by law you are to be informed of the following rights prior to interrogation:

1. You have the right remain silent. If you choose not to remain silent, anything you say can be used as evidence against you in a court of law.

2. You have a right to consult with an attorney before answering any questions and you have a right to have an attorney present during any questioning.

3. If you cannot afford an attorney, you have a right to have an attorney appointed to represent you before any questioning begins. You also have the right to have the appointed attorney present with you during such questioning.

4. You have the right to discontinue answering any questions at any time you wish.

The law further provides that any admissions made in the course of any hearing, interrogation or examination may be used as a basis for charges seeking you removal or discharge from the Department.

The undersigned hereby acknowledges that he was informed of the above rights.

Signature _____

WITNESSES

_____

_____

PREPARE IN DUPLICATE:
 Original copy to investigator's file.
 Copy to accused member

CPD-44.104 (Rev. 4/87)

COMPLAINT REGISTER NO.

ATTACHMENT NO.

"Now that you know this isn't routine anymore, can you get an attorney?"

"Oh, sure. It's part of General Order 93-3. I've got that here." She found another sheet and read, " 'Each time an interrogation is resumed, the investigator will advise the accused of the applicable criminal or statutory rights prior to the interrogation.' "

"So now you'll ask for a lawyer."

"I already have. I've told the FOP and they've assigned somebody, some guy named Quint."

"Let me get this straight. If you answer their questions, you may bring a criminal proceeding down on your head."

"Yes."

"And if you don't, they may fire you."

"Yes."

"And you still want to be a cop."

Holding her head up, she said, "It's the only thing I've ever wanted to be."

I felt very, very sorry for her. There was gallantry in her refusal to ask for sympathy. How must she feel, if she was describing the event exactly the way she remembered it, and nobody believed her? She was a lone young woman against the Chicago Police Department and the whole battery of Chicago's rapacious media.

And the situation wasn't of her making.

Frustrated for years with her sister's unholy bargain and suddenly faced with her sister stabbed, she does what she has to do. And now she's suffering for it.

"Well, even if there are discrepancies in real cases in the real world," I said, "McCoo has to come up with a narrative of the shooting that makes sense. He's on the firing line, too."

Daniello paced from the window across the room to the wall behind my chair, a distance of maybe ten feet that she covered in three strides. She paced back to the window again. She swung her arms as she walked, even though the distance was so short. Excess energy seemed to crackle out of her, from the ends of her flying hair as she turned to the tips of her spread fingers as she swung around to speak.

"What the department *could* do, if they were honest, is to ask some hard questions."

"Such as?"

She ticked them off on the fingers of her left hand, cutting at each finger with the edge of her right hand as she enumerated. "How many complaints over the years did Officer Jurack have of excessive force on the street? Not just sustained complaints, but how many complaints altogether? And where did that put him comparatively? How many CRs did he have altogether, compared to the average cop?"

"What's a CR?"

"Complaint register. You'd find him way over average. I know, because he was constantly muttering about having to put up with civilians 'bitching' about excessive force. Second—the department could check out how many times the neighbors called the cops about problems at my sister's place. Not how many times my sister actually filed a complaint, because she didn't. Twice, actually, she did, but she took it back—'failed to pursue.' If they do this—the department—they can come up with a picture of what he was really like, okay? Then they can make a real decision about whether he was the kind of guy who would attack me and whether I had to fire in self-defense. Regardless of any diddly-shit inconsistencies. Probabilities again. It's a matter of probabilities."

"But—"

"But it opens a can of worms. Every police department in this country knows that there are cops on their force that ought to be off the streets. But they're *real* slow to get rid of them. And every department in this country knows that when cops get a call to a fellow cop's house, and the wife says she's been beaten, they'll try to talk her out of filing charges. It's not just Chicago. You can bet that Spurlark would rather have the case be 'Daniello overreacts and kills brother-in-law' than

'Jurack should've been in jail, not out there roaming the streets with a badge and a gun.' "

Daniello spun around and smacked the closet door with the palm of her hand. Then she must have realized that might not be a smart way to convince me she hadn't lost her temper with Jurack. She shrugged sheepishly.

"I hated the jerk. Okay? But I didn't shoot until I was attacked. You can do the same test on me that I'm saying they should do with him. Look up my CR numbers. They're lower than average. *Lower.* I work tough, but I work smart. I don't brutalize people."

"I believe that."

"And I . . . have just got to get back on the job."

"Daniello . . ."

"Oh, shit. Call me Shelly."

Call you Superthing, I thought. But didn't say it. "And I'm Cat. Shelly, I don't know how to convince you that for both your sake and McCoo's I have to come up with a reasonable, consistent narrative of what happened. Probabilities aren't enough. People aren't predictable enough for that."

"You're not trying to pick up discrepancies? Sure you are."

"Certainly. But what I'm saying is, I'm not trying to *trap* you. I'm trying to find the areas of—of non-fit, so I can figure out where the problem is."

"You?"

"Sure. If you're telling the truth as you see it, and so are Hubner and the lab techs and the medical examiner, there's gotta be an explanation."

"I can't figure it out, and McCoo can't figure it out, the round table can't figure it out, and the IAD can't figure it out, but you're going to figure it out? Lady, you may look little, but you've got some size on you."

◆ 11 ◆

"Oh, it's *you!*" District Commander Kasmarczyk, Jurack's and Daniello's commander, looked up at me from his desk. His bushy pepper-and-salt eyebrows shaded black eyes that always looked angry. I had come to see him without asking McCoo to intercede, because I knew him. Unfortunately, he also knew me and didn't like me. There was no special reason for this; I'd always treated his people fairly when I reported on any Eighteenth District event. He just didn't like reporters.

The Eighteenth District station is located on Chicago Avenue, a few blocks west of Lake Michigan. It's an old station and it smells old. There is a story that a reporter once went to get a drink at the water fountain and roaches came out instead of water.

"Hi, Commander," I said.

"You want something on Daniello? Go to News Affairs."

"Actually, no. I want to know about Ben Jurack."

"Really? We've had about enough of that, too. Jurack was not a bad cop. I'm sick and tired of people trying to make him into Mark Fuhrman."

"No, I want to know about his day."

"What do you mean, his day?"

"The day he died. I want to know about his day here."

Kasmarczyk's eyebrows came down over his angry eyes. I was uncomfortable, but this was one thing I could do for McCoo without his help while he was recuperating.

My first instinct had been to ignore Jurack as a person and

treat him just as a piece in the puzzle. This was from a kind of prejudice that wasn't very admirable. I assumed that he was a totally rotten guy with totally rotten reasons for totally rotten behavior. So why think about him? Why pay any attention to *him* at all? But that attitude was neither fair nor thorough.

Kasmarczyk thought for half a minute. Then he said, "That's a new one." He paused. "I've had a shitload of people in here wanting to know was he this or was he that."

"By this or that you mean was he abusive to civilians?"

"That's what they wanted me to say. He wasn't. He was a good street cop. You can't treat the basic asshole crook with kid gloves. I don't know what they think we do here, escort little old ladies across the street all day? You're the first person who ever wanted to know what his day was like. Okay. You want to know, I'll tell you. But you're going to know the whole thing."

"Fine."

"I don't need some yuppie liberal acting like my men are going around hitting people right and left—"

"I'm not a yuppie. Yuppies have more money."

He almost smiled, but he remembered he didn't like me.

"Come on."

He stood up. We went out of his office, down a hall that smelled mostly of Lysol, through a locker room that smelled mostly of sweat. There were wooden benches down the middle of the locker room in front of metal lockers painted olive-green.

I said, "It looks like the locker room in a high school gym."

"Yeah, it does. This is the elegance the city of Chicago sees fit to provide its professional police officers."

"Hey, I'm reasonably sympathetic, but my profession sees fit to provide me no office at all."

"Sure. But I bet you don't spend your day dealing with drunks, child abusers, and shoplifters."

"No."

"Now follow me."

We went out the back into the parking area. We passed the spot on the building wall labeled RESERVED FOR DISTRICT COMMANDER, where his company car was parked. Next to it was a place labeled RESERVED FOR WATCH COMMANDER. Beyond that was a medium-sized lot with a mix of personal cars, squad cars, and wagons. There wasn't enough room in this lot for all the cars the district drove, and several were parked on Superior Street, some even double-parked. He found me a squad car, the nearest one. "Hop in," he said.

"Okay. Where are we going?"

"No place." He turned the car on. It smelled as if somebody had thrown up in it. Probably a drunk. Kasmarczyk said, "This here's what you might call Officer Jurack's office. Just showing you the equipment. Now, this is a new car. Not bad, huh? Now watch."

He flicked on the heater. "Nothing, right?" he said. "Heater gave up two weeks ago and the city hasn't fixed it yet. Take a look at the back seat."

"Cut up some," I said.

"Yup. They haul around people who think it's proper revenge to take their frustrations out on the upholstery. Talented, too. They can rip up a seat with their fingernails when their hands are handcuffed behind their backs. Never think if they hadn't held up the currency exchange they might not be in the back of a squad car. Elegant it isn't. You agree?"

"Sure. But it's not so terrible, either."

"Good cop, Jurack. He saw a problem, he'd take care of it. You could always count on him to pick up a speeder. Not like some guys, they want to avoid the paper. Didn't bother him. Now follow me."

Back in his office, Kasmarczyk said, "I looked up his day myself after he died. It went like this. He was working six A.M. to two P.M. Which meant he was an early car on that shift. You know we have early cars and late cars on every tour, so there's always somebody on the streets to protect and serve the citizenry?"

"I knew that."

Kasmarczyk held several sheets of paper which he barely glanced at. "So, first thing out he had two parking violations. Six-thirty A.M. Early morning, businesses starting to open up, one of them a restaurant, they find somebody parking where they need to get their deliveries in. You know."

"Yeah. Okay."

"I can tell you from experience, they want you to tow that car instantly. They find you need to call for a tow and it takes time, they get angry. Like the city of Chicago has thousands of tow trucks, one waiting right outside their store."

"Okay, I get the picture."

"Then he had a truancy. Kid did not arrive at school. Parents had been warned. Kid had been warned yay times. Jurack went to the home. The kid screamed and yelled at him. Then both the parents screamed and yelled at him."

"Who did you find this out from? His partner?"

"No. One of the parents came in here and complained. Jurack didn't have a partner. He was a ninety-nine unit."

"Did Jurack not have a partner because he was too angry and too difficult to work with?"

"I'm not going to reply to that."

Which of course meant yes. "Go ahead."

"By then the stores were open. As you probably know, the Eighteenth District covers some of the most unlivable public housing in Chicago and also the Gold Coast and the 'Magnificent Mile'—Bloomie's, Neiman Marcus, Lord and Taylor, Armani."

"I knew that."

"A fun district, huh? Variety. Anyhow, next he got a shoplifter call. And whattaya know. It's an alderman's wife. She has three very heavy gold necklaces in her purse, tags still on them, she's found halfway out the door of a store whose name you would instantly recognize but I'm not gonna mention, and the sales clerk absolutely furious, partly because she just told him she wouldn't put one of those necklaces on her dog—which she said was an apricot poodle—because they were so ugly, and while he goes to get something else for her to look at, she steals them. So Jurack arrests her. She's screaming. The clerk and store manager are not quite screaming, but they're speaking very, very tight-throated. And *then the alderman arrives!*"

"I get the picture."

"The whole shootin' match, even the clerk, gets brought over here."

"Right."

"And they all tell me exactly how they feel about it. After we sort all that out, Jurack goes to early lunch. There's a restaurant on Chestnut gives cops free lunches as long as they come in at non-busy hours. They especially like having them there at night. Keeps the assholes from shooting up the place, locking the staff in the refrigerator, killing everybody, you know."

"Yes."

"So he's eating lunch minding his own business, and they have a disturbance with a drunk. Well, that's pretty much what he's there for, so he has to handle it, right in the middle of his steak and eggs."

"Right."

"That was just before eleven. Now he's back on the job. Grabs a speeder on State Street. Can you imagine doing fifty on State Street in the middle of the day? You can kill a hundred and seventeen people per block. And that's why Jurack was so good. He'd see something like that, he'd go after them. Wasn't worried about the paperwork, he'd go after them. He's the cop the good citizen *wants* out there."

"I hear you."

"Then he had a call of a bum on Michigan Avenue accosting people. People don't like that. They're on their way to buy their Godiva chocolates at Water Tower Place, some bum is wiping dirty hands on their Guccis."

"Right."

"Bum swore at him, but Jurack wouldn't be bothered by

that. Arrested him. Asshole threw up in his car. Then he got a false holdup alarm from the Walgreen's. Then he got his last call of the day. Neighbor calling about child abuse, we call it a child-endangerment call. He goes over to Evergreen. Turns out to be two children. Garbage in the apartment is up to his hips. Baby in a diaper that had not been changed in days. You could smell the kid from the hall outside, which is why the neighbor called the cops. Kid's screaming. Sores all over the kid's bottom from the piss and shit. Three-year-old girl eating dog food, but no dog in the apartment and no mother or father either. Jurack sends for the evidence tech for pictures. He sends for the Department of Children and Family Services to come for the kids. He sends for a supervisor. All the right things. What with one thing and another, this takes him a little past the end of his tour, which is two o'clock. Two-fifteen he's leaving the building right behind the DCFS people, and from one of the windows up in the building, fourth or fifth floor maybe, somebody pisses on him."

"Oh, my God."

"Right. Oh, my God. Lucky he was wearing his cap. Jurack doesn't even go back in to see who it was. Coulda been anybody and there's no fingerprints on piss. He comes back here, takes his uniform off to get it cleaned, makes out his reports. Gets done about forty minutes past the end of his shift. And then we let him go home."

"I hear what you're saying."

"Did he keep some people from getting run down by a car? Did he save a little kid's life? Who knows? Did his day make him irritable? Who knows? If it did, should it have? Would it have made you irritable? Who knows? He put in his eight hours, plus a little, and then we let him go home."

I got a full night's sleep, and for the first time in more than a week I slept at the time normal people do—nighttime. I woke up Friday morning bursting with energy and ready to right all the world's wrongs, or at least whichever of them took place east of State Street, west of Holden Court, south of Eighth, and north of Twelfth.

Heading out my building's front door, I almost stepped on my landlord, Mr. Whillis. Mr. Whillis is approximately fifty-five, has thinning reddish hair, and doesn't look too bad. On the outside. On the inside he's slimy green, with fangs, and a gaping, hungry maw surrounded by sharp, snaggly teeth.

"Did you get my message, Miss Marsala?"

"Uh, yes, I did." I thought of lying. Decided to start the day right for a change.

"I'll need your decision, Miss Marsala. Do you plan to stay on?"

"Mr. Whillis, are you planning to fix that window where the water comes in and leaks across the sill?"

"I suppose I'd have to if I were showing the apartment to a prospective new tenant . . ."

"Suppose you think of me as an old tenant who is thinking about becoming a prospective new tenant?"

He smiled, a nasty smile. "So you plan to stay?"

"I have to check my budget, Mr. Whillis. I'm not sure I can afford the higher rent."

"Let me know . . ."

"And I'm sure it will be a serious hardship for Mr. Ederle." My downstairs neighbor, old and on a fixed income.

"Miss Marsala, the higher real estate taxes are a hardship for me. Changing all the paperwork is very burdensome. Nor will I emerge from this with any additional money, I assure you. Research the tax changes if you doubt my word. I hear you're quite the little researcher."

"I'll let you know, Mr. Whillis."

"By the end of the month, Miss Marsala."

Taxes had gone up. That was no lie. I hate it when people I don't like have some good reasons on their side.

Speaking of money and higher rent, six weeks earlier I had done a story, a profile on the founder of the Upper Avenue

Improv Theater, for *Chicago Faces*. The check should have
arrived by now. What had arrived instead in yesterday's mail,
which I got around to reading over breakfast, was a notice
that *Chicago Faces* had gone out of business. The money
wouldn't be forthcoming. And it was remarkably nice of them
even to spend a stamp to tell the contributors that much. A lot
of magazines folded in total silence.

I was not letting any of this depress me. It was time to get
to McCoo's office and mount our counterattack. Never mind
that it was only eight forty-five. Somewhere out in space I
picked up what McCoo would be saying at the hospital: "You
told me I'd get out today, and it's today and I'm leaving!"

The nurse says, "You have to be discharged, sir. Your doctor
will be here soon."

"And I'll be out of here now. Susanne, hand me my pants."

Susanne says, "Harold, please . . ."

The nurse says, "Sir . . ."

McCoo says, "Quarter of nine! I haven't got to the office
this late in years."

Was I ever right. At three minutes before nine, carrying my
surprise package, which had been X-rayed by the guard at the
entrance, I got into the elevator at Eleventh and State, the big
cop shop. Fred Koy stepped on behind me. We quick-walked
around the corner on eight to the chief of detectives' office.
McCoo was already there, standing in the middle of the main
room, staring down at the burned area on the floor. As we
walked in, he hastily looked away from the damage. By the
time Fred and I had put our coats in the little cupboard, Russell Lupinski had come off another elevator. Russell also
glanced at the place where Bramble's desk had been.

"Russell, you look awful," McCoo said.

"You don't look so great either, boss."

"I'm fine. I'm just fine."

I said to Russell, "What did they do to you?" The entire

right side of his head was bandaged. Unlike McCoo. McCoo's hair had been shaved on one side, but the bandages were gone.

Just then Tracy Shoemaker entered. It was now one minute short of nine and everybody was here. McCoo runs a tight ship. Like the rest of us, she let her gaze slip to the burned area, then turned away.

Russell said, "I didn't hurt my head. My head's too hard. But I'm gonna look like Mr. Spock when this bandage comes off."

"You lost your ear?"

"A little slice off the back. Like I said, I'll look like Spock. I'm gonna have a pointed ear."

McCoo went to his office, but the door was locked. "What the hell—" he said.

Tracy said, "Oh. Right. When the ATF—"

Koy said, "—and the bomb squad left, they locked the door. You're supposed to call Security—"

"—to bring you your key," Tracy said, grabbing the phone.

McCoo growled, "Damn! Yeah, now that you remind me, my key was in my desk drawer. I never went back to get it after the blast." He folded his arms impatiently, but in fact he only had a couple of minutes to rumble and mutter before the key came and he went into his office to see what the damage looked like.

Koy said to Russell, "Well, at least you didn't miss work."

I said, "What do you mean? Of course he missed work."

"No, yesterday was his off day. We rotate."

"Because somebody has to be in the office on Saturday and Sunday," Koy said. "So one week I have Monday off and take Saturday and Russell has Tuesday off and gets Sunday, and the next week Tracy does Saturday and I do Sunday, and so on. See?"

"Oh. Didn't Bramble do a day?" I thought bringing her name up would be healthful for everybody. We'd been pussyfooting around it for too long.

"Bramble *assigned* the days. She didn't take the weekends.

But actually she did more work than the rest of us. She was on call. Nights, weekends, holidays."

Tracy said, "She and the boss both carry beepers—carried beepers—twenty-four hours."

Koy said, "And if anybody couldn't get the boss by phone for an emergency, they'd call Bramble."

Tracy said, "Uh—you know the funeral isn't set yet. They may need more tissue samples than they—"

There was a bellow from McCoo's office. We ran.

"Boss!" Lupinski said. "Are you hurt?"

"Look at that!" McCoo pointed at his coffeemaker, with its cracked carafe. "Look at that!"

"Uh-oh!" Tracy said.

"Ha!" I said.

Fred said, "Ha what?"

"Thought of it on my way home last night. My way home leads past Marshall Field. Take a look in here."

He opened my package. A new carafe.

With real admiration in his voice, Russell Lupinski said, "Good move, Marsala."

Then the place really started to hum. A pair of detectives arrived at the moment McCoo was having Russell send for three more. McCoo had assigned the two from his hospital bed to canvass all the offices on this floor and ask whether anybody saw any strangers hanging around. Now he said, "Go back and get a narration of everything anybody noticed in the halls that whole morning. And write it down! I don't care how minor it sounds." The two detectives nodded but looked uncomfortable; I suppose they were used to doing that kind of work out in a neighborhood, not right here in the CPD.

McCoo had Tracy call the lab, to ask whether the envelope had been reconstructed yet. "And tell them I want to know whether it came through the post office, or the CPD mail, or was just dropped here."

"Sure, boss."

"And by the way, I want the three of you to sit down and write out everybody you saw in the office or in the hall that morning."

"Right, boss."

McCoo had Fred call the area commander, who technically would be in charge of the detectives on all cases that happened in this district. Between them, they would parcel out the work of solving Bramble's murder. Since McCoo was the superior officer, parceling that out would be nothing compared to the difficulties of dealing with the feds.

"How do you divide the responsibilities between ATF and the CPD?"

"It's worse than a negotiation at Camp David."

"But how?"

"They'd just better realize I'm in charge," he said.

"And they'll accept that? Isn't that expecting too much?"

"It's optimistic. But it better work."

I trekked back with McCoo into his office.

There were three or four piles of papers and envelopes that the techs and ATF people and so on must have brought in here yesterday from the outer office. Some piles had scorched edges and there were several sheets of paper that were half burned. Ash and chunks of black paper littered his floor.

I said, "Do we assume Bomb and Arson has finished with this stuff?"

"Oh, they'd take what they wanted to look at, you can bet on that. Especially ATF. These are not shy, retiring guys."

"Yeah. They'd take whatever told them something about the physical nature of the bomb. But the reason for the blast might be in here."

"The reason for the blast was me."

"You think they wanted to kill you?"

"Sure. Don't you?"

"Yes, probably. The envelope was addressed to you. But suppose you weren't the target? For instance, suppose instead they wanted to destroy all of that day's mail?"

"Possible. We should go through all these papers."

I was pleased that he said "we." "Do we know what we're looking for?"

"No."

"You want to start now?"

I looked at his face and realized how weary he was. McCoo was not a well man, however much he pretended to be okay. And I wasn't ready to take a chance of damaging wet papers, not knowing what we were looking for. Sighing, he said, "No. Not at all, really. But we better not lose anything. I'll lock this stuff in my safe."

"Excellent."

We shoved all the papers in McCoo's rather small office safe. Fortunately, there wasn't such a lot of it. It was mainly the leftovers of mail and paperwork that had been in and around Bramble's smashed desk, after the various agencies had taken the desk and the suspicious elements of the bomb away.

When we finished, I said, "I talked with Shelly Daniello."

"And?"

"I like her. And she talks well. But I don't know whether to believe her or not. She's convincing, in the sense that her behavior and personality are all of a piece. She's smart. Competent. Tough. Angry, but not crazy with anger."

"She's got a good record."

"I know. Now I'd like to see Jurack's work history. Daniello mentioned it."

"No problem. Ask Fred. He does most of our Personnel records. Did Daniello explain the discrepancies in her story any better?"

"No. A little fuller narration. But the three serious discrepancies are still there. I want to go to the ME and find out exactly when he thinks that bruise on the head happened. 'Around the time of death' is too vague."

"Okay. Yeah, it would help if it was during Jurack's fight with his wife, which makes sense to me."

"Jurack did not fight with his wife, McCoo. Jurack beat his wife."

"Sorry. You know what I mean."

"Anyhow, I agree she might have hit him back. If somebody was coming after me with a knife, I'd hit him with anything I had handy."

"Point taken, Cat."

"So can you can get the ME to talk to me?"

"Easily."

"McCoo, what do you think about Daniello's claim that when she fired she was several feet from Jurack?"

"The lab says no. That's one of the main reasons they think she's lying. The powder marks are so definite. But you know, that was one of the reasons I believed her in the first place."

"Why? Spell this one out for me."

"Somebody's coming at you with a knife. First choice: You fire when he's four feet away. Second choice: You wait until he's almost on top of you and then you fire. Which makes you look better, if you're a cop?"

"Wait until he's on top of you, of course. It looks like you did everything else you could, first. Yelled or whatever."

"You showed restraint."

"Sure. Plus Jurack is more of a threat at one foot than four feet."

He said, "Especially in an emotionally charged situation like this. Your brother-in-law has stabbed your sister? I mean, come on!" He lightened his voice a bit, to imitate Shelly's: " 'I didn't want to shoot him, Commander. The knife was almost at my throat when I finally had to fire.' "

I said, "So why didn't she say that?"

He said, "My point exactly. It's like an 'admission against interest' in court. It's like the chunk of ice in her other case. I think it was because she was telling the truth."

◇ 12 ◇

Dr. Suvitha, who had done the autopsy, would not be in until afternoon. McCoo promised he would call the Medical Examiner's Office again right after lunch to make sure Suvitha would see me.

Another three detectives turned up. They were part of a four-person task force McCoo had assigned to work directly with the Bomb and Arson and ATF people, who were mainly finding and analyzing the explosive material and bomb parts. They wanted to report how the "liaising" was working out. Since there was no way that McCoo could pass me off as any sort of police officer or legitimate investigator, he waved a dismissive hand at me, swept the three men into his office, and closed the door behind himself.

The best thing to do with the rest of the morning was run down one of the top cops and grill him. Subtly. McCoo couldn't make this contact for me, of course, because we didn't want the top cop even to know I was friends with McCoo. Besides which, with McCoo twisting in the wind right now, they would probably want to distance themselves from him. I had with me a letter from Hal explaining the type of article I was doing, rather carefully vague in its phrasing:

> CHICAGO TODAY is planning an article or series of articles on the upper echelons of the Chicago Police Department. If you could give our reporter, Catherine Marsala, any assistance, we would certainly be grateful.
>
> Hal Briskman, Managing Editor, *Chicago Today*

This note cleverly did not say whether we were doing the top cops themselves or the department as a whole. Or whether we were doing one top cop or all of them. With the impending mayoral election and political shake-ups, each of our targets would probably salivate at the chance of getting press coverage. Being known favorably to the public couldn't hurt in the selection process. The whiff of "gratitude" at the end of Hal's missive hinted at, but did not promise, some support or at least some inches of copy during the coming upheaval.

Well done, Hal. But whether it would work we would soon see.

The various floors of the CPD building at Eleventh and State have distinct personalities. The second floor, which houses the Crime Lab, Ballistics, and other such scientific pursuits, has a businesslike rustle, occasional laughter, not a whole lot of urgency. The eighth floor, where the Personnel Office, McCoo's office, and a couple of courtrooms, including one affectionately known as hooker court, are located, has an interesting mixture of efficiency and desperation about it. The third and fourth floors, which contain the radio dispatchers and 911 banks, are entirely different from the others. Exterior corridors run around inner walls of glass. Through these indoor windows you can look down onto rank after rank of dispatchers sitting at command modules and facing elaborate maps of the part of the city they watch over.

The top-cops floor, the fifth, is entirely different. Here uniformed cops walk softly, speak carefully, and wear all parts of their uniform in spick-and-span order at all times. Chicago pols, however, stride along casually and guffaw as often as possible, trying to imply that they own somebody in one of the command offices. The fifth floor is the floor of camel-hair topcoats and Italian silk neckties.

Start at the top, I thought, as I got out of the elevator on the fifth floor.

*　　　*　　　*

All happy police departments resemble each other. Each unhappy police department is unhappy in its own way. New York has been tainted repeatedly with corruption. Los Angeles has to deal with a subgroup of jackbooted thugs.

Chicago's particular source of unhappiness is too much politics. Politics in hiring. Politics in promotions. Politics in picking the top cops.

A police department is a semimilitary organization. Or militaroid. Whatever. They have a similar command structure, with patrol officers out in the trenches, and ranks through sergeant, lieutenant, up to the general at the top. In Chicago, unlike a lot of cities, the general is not called the chief of police but the superintendent of police. The structure, however, remains the same. Orders come from the top down and obedience from the bottom up, as in an army. But a police department is not an army. Police officers are not really involved in a war, no matter how often the media call it that, and they are not an occupying army, either. Many a police department has gotten into serious trouble for treating the populace as the enemy.

Above the superintendent is the de facto head of the police, the mayor of Chicago.

Days away from a mayoral election is fear-and-trembling time for the Chicago Police Department. At normal times, people know where they stand. There are shake-ups, sure, but people have some idea where they'll come from. From the top. Now the top itself could be shaken up. Would be.

In the ordinary course of events, a reporter applies to the News Affairs Office to get permission to do a story on some aspect of the department. News Affairs then lets the target group—say it's the Crime Lab—know whether or not they are permitted to cooperate with the reporter.

Sometimes a reporter will approach the police officers directly. The officers then call News Affairs and get permission. If they're smart.

When top cops are approached by reporters, they will ordinarily check with the superintendent unless it's a routine matter.

Not now.

With the election hanging over everybody's head, the four deputy superintendents knew that Superintendent Spurlark wouldn't demote any of them; making any big changes now would give the impression that his original appointee had not been well chosen. And now the top cops themselves were all jockeying for attention, not with the superintendent, but with the outside world. They might very well want to talk with me.

I went into the anteroom of the superintendent's suite. The large paneled office was crowded with news people eager for a follow-up on the bombing. I knew most of them. I wasn't doing the bombing as a story and really did not want to be associated with it. I stopped before anybody saw me and backed out.

Across from the superintendent's office was the office of Gregory Dennison Winter. Deputy Superintendent Winter headed the Bureau of Technical Services, supervising the Communications Division, General Support, Records, and the Crime Lab. Each of these divisions had its own commander, who reported directly to Winter.

Winter was the guy McCoo had called "real smart." Winter was also the guy he said had gone to law school and had a rich family. McCoo said, "Everything has always come easy to Winter."

Well, we'd just see.

And we did. In two minutes I was back in the hall.

Winter's office had been guarded by a very small woman, a white lady with black eyes, plum-colored hair, and a pointed chin. She was tiny. Arms like pencils and a body not much thicker than a two-quart Diet Pepsi bottle.

Her manner was enough to make up for her size.

"Deputy Superintendent Winter is far too busy to see anyone this morning."

Past her, in the inner office, I saw Winter's assistant deputy
superintendent at a desk, studying papers. Ordinary eight-
and-a-half-by-eleven-inch sheets of paper that must be
reports and letters. But beyond him, in the inner-inner office,
Gregory Dennison Winter stood at a window intently studying a newspaper.

Busy indeed!

I had explained to bird lady that I was a reporter for
Chicago Today, that I was doing a series of articles on the
upper echelons of the department. I said *"Chicago Today"*
quite loudly, and had the satisfaction of seeing Winter's head
rise just a fraction of an inch, but he didn't come running out.
Bird lady took my card and promised she would "query
Deputy Superintendent Winter when he becomes available."

Thinking, Winter, you ought to keep your door closed, I left.

Twenty feet down the hall was the office of First Deputy
Superintendent Robert Cleary. This was my fourth office visit
of the morning, if you counted McCoo's. I fully expected to
be going in and out of offices all day, if not all week, sort of the
Flying Dutchman of the Chicago Police Department.

"My name is Cat Marsala," I said to Cleary's civilian secretary in the outer-outer office. Cleary's door guardian was not
small and birdlike. He was a tall black man with a scholarly
face. Sitting down, he was as tall as I was standing. His only
similarity to the bird lady was that he was very slender.

"I'm a reporter for *Chicago Today*. I'm doing a story on the
upper echelons of the Chicago Police Department—"

"Miss Marsala!" a voice boomed from the back regions. The
secretary blinked wearily, which was his only show of emotion.

Doing a ninety-degree turn fast, I saw a hand thrust out at
me and a big pink face smiling happily. He grabbed my hand
before I could even raise it, and squeezed.

"I'm Bob Cleary!" he said, in a voice that made his poor
secretary blink again. "Come on in!"

Isn't that the way? Just when you think you have a real struggle ahead—

Cleary headed the Bureau of Operational Services. The divisions under him were Patrol, Traffic, and Operations Command, each of which was headed by its own commander. As first dep, Cleary was a big enchilada, second only to the superintendent.

"Sit down! Sit down! Tell me about your project! I've seen your byline, haven't I?"

"Well, you may have. I work freelance for several papers and magazines. I did a major story on level-one trauma units recently that you might have seen—"

"I did see it! You were absolutely right. We have to find some new ways to pay for trauma units. We can't count on the hospitals' being willing to lose money on them! No wonder they close down."

"Actually, I didn't take sides." How could McCoo be best buddies with this glad-handing loudmouth? How could McCoo and his plump, pretty, fierce, no-nonsense wife enjoy going out to dinner once a month with this guy? This was the type of guy who would call a waitress "honey."

But I stopped myself right there. I realized I couldn't tell what Cleary was really like. I was an outsider. To most cops all noncops are outsiders, and cops put on a public face.

"So, what I can help you with?" Cleary boomed.

I showed him my letter from Hal, which he waved away as if my honesty were written right above my nose. I said, "The present police administration will be taking the department into the twenty-first century, and they'll—"

"That's a very good way to put it! But any improvements we expect to have in place for the next century, we definitely have to start now. You can't decide in the year 2000 that you're going to make earth-shattering improvements," he said at ear-shattering volume.

And he was off at top speed, telling me about his grandfather, from Back-of-the-Yards, who was a cop in the days when "there were no radios, no nothing; you cranked call boxes at certain locations on your beat. They couldn't have *imagined* handheld radios for every officer." This launched him into an impassioned discussion of the need for a new headquarters building "with all the power cables for electronic assistance built in from the git-go." Apparently we especially needed heavy-duty cabling for a computer-aided dispatch system, without which we could not hold our heads up in the latter part of the twentieth century, let alone setting foot in the twenty-first.

His big pink face glistened with a light sheen of sweat. He was chubby, and the face was round as a pink moon, eyes stretched horizontal by his round cheeks, mouth stretched out in a perpetual smile. I took notes carefully, schizoid with trying both to study his facial expressions and write at the same time. Being a belt-plus-suspenders type as far as my work was concerned, I had also laid my small tape recorder on his desk and turned it on, making an eyebrows-up gesture to him, so as not to stop the flow of words. He airily waved his permission at it and went on without losing momentum.

As he segued into a description of his two lovely daughters and two handsome sons, I looked around his office. There were five—count 'em, five—pictures of the Saint Patrick's Day Parade. In four of them he was marching next to Mayor Richard M. Daley. In another photo, in living color, he was at some sort of green-beer gala, wearing a green top hat which looked Christmassy next to his red face, round as a glass ornament. In a black-and-white photo, a portly Cleary look-alike shook hands with John Fitzgerald Kennedy. Bob Cleary's father, I was sure. There was another photo of the father with Richard J. Daley, locally known as Daley the First. All we needed was a bumper sticker saying "Kiss me, I'm Irish."

He moved smoothly into ten minutes of campaign promises, only lightly disguised as telling me about himself. He made sure he slowed down enough for me to write down every precious word. Did he want to be superintendent? Oh, my, did he! Finally, he had covered everything he could think of and regretfully ground to a stop.

He leaned closer to me and spoke confidentially. "If I'm gonna talk straight with you, I'd like to be able to see the article before it comes out."

"Okay."

"Okay?" He was surprised, as well he might be. Reporters are a hard-bitten lot. But I didn't care; I wanted him loose and happy.

"Yeah. It's okay. I told you, I'm doing a profile. Not an exposé."

"Sure. That's great. Well, Cat, it's like this. The public really *wants* police officers who are tough on the street. They want cops to come down hard when they see bunches of teenage boys hanging around the corner. Gangs like that *scare* older people."

"But a bunch of kids hanging around a street corner after school isn't necessarily a gang."

"Of course not. But the old fo——senior citizens—don't care whether these kids are affiliated with some gang or whether they're just a bunch of bored kids who want to trip up elderly people and take their purses and wallets. *They want them out of there.* They want them sent home."

He went on. "Your good citizens don't care if the police bust into some drug house without knocking. The public doesn't give a—uh, doesn't care beans about the Constitution unless it's them that get busted in on, and they figure it won't be. They want tough cops! When I was first on the job we were expected to administer a little street justice. A cop had to be as tough as the crooks, but on the right side of the law."

The glad-hander had now metamorphosed into something quite different. An old, angry beat cop. I could picture him on the street, billy club in hand. I decided he was not only tougher, but smarter than he looked.

I said, "But these days you're getting a more educated recruit, aren't you?"

"And paying more. A cop today makes good money."

I decided to give him a shot. "Not like the days when Daley the First said you don't have to pay cops much because they can steal?"

"Mmmm. Yes. Less enlightened times. Less enlightened times. He had his faults, but he was a great mayor for this city."

"And now you have—what is it?—twenty-five, thirty percent women cops, too?"

"Mmmm. Right." His grudging tone said it all. But he was too canny to get drawn into a discussion of females on the force with a female reporter.

I said, pushing him, "The Shelly Daniello thing. Certainly that case isn't typical of female cops?"

He eyed me sharply. "This going to be in your story?"

"No, it is not. I'm doing a profile, pure and simple."

"I'll tell you one thing. Our chief of detectives, Harold McCoo, is the best in the business. I don't know this Officer Daniello personally, but I can tell you everything about McCoo. He's an old-line, solid, smart detective with decades of experience. And he's an honest man. If he says Daniello's story smells right to him, then it's right. And much as I admire Chicago's fine cadre of reporters, you haven't treated McCoo well."

"It wasn't me—"

"I'm not saying you personally. But the interest of the media isn't in justice, it's in a story. They don't care whose career they destroy."

"They try to verify that the source—"

"Do they? Do they always? Do they all?"

"Uh, no, not all. But the good ones—"

"You ask me, the good ones are rare. Anyhow." He took a breath and whooshed out a big gust of air. "I got a meeting to go to."

"Oh. Okay." I stood up. "I really appreciate this—"

"Now, you said you'd send me the article to approve ahead of publication."

"And I meant it. We're talking publication tomorrow morning, so I'll be working on it this evening. I could fax it to you by nine tonight." No way I could get it done earlier, if I was going to go to the medical examiner after lunch.

"Well, I don't know—"

"Do you have a fax at home?"

"No. Ought to get one."

"In your office?"

"No."

"I see." That meant it was in the general office somewhere, and he was worried somebody there could read what I had written and know he was in on the approval of it.

He brightened. "I could send an officer to your place to get a copy."

"Fine with me. Say nine P.M.?" I gave him my address.

"Franklin Street, huh? I had a beat there when I was just a rookie."

"Well, thank you for the information. I hope you like the result. I assume *Chicago Today* has a photo of you?"

"Yeah. They've got a recent one."

"Great. That's it, then."

"You're okay, Miss Marsala. But you tell your colleagues they pick on McCoo, they're picking on the wrong person."

· 13 ·

"Your friend not coming to lunch with you?" Hermione said. I was hungry and needed really hot chili or a big bowl of soup. It was past the worst of the lunch rush, and Hermione steered me toward a table near the front window.

"My friend?"

"The one who liked my chocolate cheesecake."

I started to say everybody liked her chocolate cheesecake, when I realized. *Bramble.* I had been here only the day before yesterday with Bramble. So many things had happened, it seemed as if it had been two weeks ago.

Hermione must have noticed that I went blank, because she asked, "You two have a fight? You're not bringing her back?"

"I'm not bringing her back," I said, and tears filled my eyes.

"Uh-oh," Hermione said. "I think my office is a better place for your lunch."

"Oh, God, I thought I was over this."

She sat me down in a wonderful overstuffed, rump-sprung chair in a space the size of a large broom closet. There were actually several brooms and a vacuum in the corner. Hermione believes in using restaurant space for tables or for cooking, not for her own comfort.

"So tell," she said, and I told her.

When I finished she just nodded and left. Half a minute later she was back. "Here's soup."

"I'm not as hungry as I thought I was."

"Eat. It's my Dutch treat. Wednesdays only. Dutch pea

soup redolent—yes, I said redolent—of ham bits and mett-
wurst."

Fragrant steam rose up around me.

"Eat," Hermione said. Hermione is one of those lucky people who went into exactly the right line of work.

"Eat," she repeated.

"Well, maybe just a taste."

She smiled.

"You have to understand capillaries," Dr. Emmy Suvitha said.

"Yes?"

"You give someone a sharp blow. Like this." She snapped
the edge of her stapler down hard on her desk. I jumped.
Suvitha was a delicate-boned, gentle-looking woman, and the
crack surprised me.

"Now if this were human skin instead of a plastic desktop,"
she said, "what would start happening? Blood would begin to
leak from the damaged capillaries. Assuming you had not
actually lacerated a larger vein or artery—and usually you
don't; they're pretty tough—the leak would be fairly slow.
Small vessels, do you see?"

"Yes, I think so."

"Both blood cells and fluid, serum, would leak. The area
would slowly start to swell and discolor. Slowly."

"Yes. How slowly?"

"Well, of course, that is the question. Your Mr. Jurack, now,
if we had him in front of us you would see for yourself, this
forehead blow was not hard enough to break the skin. Not a
fierce blow. So now you have blood leaking from damaged
capillaries, under the pressure of the heart. The blood pressure, you see?"

"Yes."

"If the heart stops, no pressure. Or usually no pressure. In
the old days, pathologists would sometimes make terribly
erroneous estimates of the severity of a blow when they

examined embalmed bodies. If the investigator did not see the body until after it had been embalmed, the bruising would look much worse than it really was, because the embalming fluid is forced in under pressure and it pushes more blood out of the damaged vessels."

"I see."

"Not the case here, of course."

"No."

"It is the red cells that cause the most discoloration. That is what makes what you call a bruise."

Suvitha's desk held photos of three children. A single picture showed two girls who looked like twins. Another was a boy about ten in white shirt and a narrow tie around a long, thin neck. When I arrived at the medical examiner's office, Dr. Suvitha had been eating a lunch packed in a metal Casper the Friendly Ghost lunch box. People are always amazed that a doctor can go from an autopsy to lunch and back to another autopsy after lunch. What do they expect? Pathologists get hungry, just like other people.

"So this bruise . . ."

She said, "Leaving aside embalming, when the heart stops, the pressure stops, and there is no more swelling or discoloration of the ecchymoses. In this case, very, very little swelling or leakage had occurred before the heart stopped. One can see the mark on the skin, yes. One can see the damage microscopically as well. But it had not advanced very far."

"How far? How long had it been?"

"It is very difficult to tell whether a bruise was made within a minute or two before death to a few seconds after. There still is some residual pressure, you see."

"Then you're saying this blow to the head came right around his death?"

"Exactly."

"Could it have been made three minutes before?"

"Possibly."

"Ten minutes?"

"I do not think so."

"Not twenty, then? Or thirty?" Ben Jurack had been beating his wife, Marie, for at least half an hour. He was dead by the time the EMTs got through their examination of him on the floor of the television room, even though they took him to the trauma unit, where a doctor formally pronounced him dead. At the time the EMTs arrived, Shelly Daniello had been in the house fifteen minutes at the very most.

Suvitha said, "Definitely no. There is not enough discoloration or swelling. The man was struck just minutes before death or moments after."

So Marie Jurack did not hit him during the earlier "fight." And Shelly Daniello could have hit him. With her gun?

"What sort of thing made the wound, Dr. Suvitha?"

"It is just an edge. Not a sharp edge, not like a metal ruler or the edge of a piece of wood. Not quite as sharp as the edge on this stapler. But an edge nevertheless."

"A long thing?"

"I do not know. See my forehead? Now look." She held a ruler up next to it. "One's head is rounded, you see, so if it is hit by a straight weapon, not much of the weapon actually contacts the head. Do you understand what I mean? The bruise on Mr. Jurack is just slightly over an inch long. It could have been made by almost anything."

"Could it have been the side of an automatic, a gun? They have squarish barrels."

"It certainly could."

I met John for dinner, and by then I really needed coddling. John Banks, my semi-significant other, is a stockbroker who spends some of his time helping the firm bring out new companies, getting financing, writing public-offering documents. As if he didn't make serious money himself, his parents are loaded. They live in one of those tall houses on narrow lots next to the lake north of Streeterville, which is the beginning of Chicago's Gold Coast. The house has three stories, not counting the basement, and is made of granite blocks the size of Toyotas.

The trouble with the Banks family is a certain pervasive dullness. Mrs. Banks considers pizza an extremely exotic food, eaten by immigrants and by people who don't have the sense not to be gastronomically adventurous. Mr. Banks is the kind of man who would wear a dark-blue-and-gray paisley tie in the shower, if he could avoid getting it wet.

John himself is a truly nice man. He is even sensitive, often giving me a present that is precisely what I need. But not exactly romantic. One birthday, when Mr. Whillis was being a particularly nasty landlord, John gave me a new toilet.

Tonight he took me to Le Perroquet. Oh, my! Lovely food. No better than Hermione's, really, but lovely. Peppery watercress soup. Beef bourguignonne that was delicate but rich. A red wine like a distilled sunset.

He told me about his experiences in Hong Kong. His firm was "bringing out" a women's clothing company devoted, as best I could understand it, entirely to luxurious silks.

He asked what I had been doing. I explained that I had to get home right after dinner to finish writing the first of the deputy superintendent profiles. I'd gotten about two hours of work in on it before meeting John. And I explained why I was writing them.

"Cat, this isn't going to work for you."

"What do you mean?"

He spread sweet butter on a piece of crusty roll.

"Four small articles about the top cops isn't going to pay your rent."

"Well, of course not. But I have to do it for McCoo."

"Sure, but what are you accomplishing, really? I don't see how you can figure anything out about that unfortunate shooting that he and the police lab can't figure out for themselves."

"Well, I might. But he also wants me to assess Montoya, Winter, Cleary, and Bannister."

"Which will be useless."

"What do you mean?"

"You can talk to them, and you may distrust one more than the others. In fact, statistically I suppose you will necessarily distrust one more than the others. But so what?"

"Then I'll tell McCoo."

"But don't you see? You won't *know* anything. It's silly. You can't actually tell who is masterminding the leaks to the press. There's just no way to be sure of a thing like that. There aren't any 'clues.'"

"McCoo needs help. He needs to feel somebody is on his side. I may not be able to figure everything out myself, but we can pool what we know—"

"McCoo is asking the impossible."

"Not entirely impossible—"

"And he's not being fair to you. You need to keep your mind on your career."

I stared at John. "Unless," he added in a firm tone, "you would agree to marry me."

I've turned him down three times. I said, "Not now, John. I can't get into this right now."

"Then you have to protect yourself. Tell McCoo you have your own work to do. Explain to him what he's asking is impossible."

"McCoo is my friend. I have to do whatever I can."

"He's asking too much."

"John, McCoo is a good man. He's just *such* a good man. Not once in all of this mess has he taken the easy way. Not once has he suggested lying about the facts, to Daniello or me or anybody. He may not be thinking clearly. Partly that's because these are his friends, people whose histories and daily problems he understands. But *still* his basic good character comes through. He won't sacrifice anybody for his own skin. He could easily have thrown Daniello to the wolves. Or—just think of the number of ways he could fudge or fabricate evidence! He could get somebody to testify falsely, by promising advancement or money. In his position he could actually fake documents or evidence. He could get out of this even now by abandoning Daniello."

"I'm sure he's a good man. I never said he wasn't. I'm only saying you have to think of yourself."

"He's my friend. I can't walk away from him."

"I guess it's your funeral."

Lately, we always end up arguing.

· 14 ·

I lay in a sea of bubbles.

Only seconds had passed between the departure of the messenger from Cleary and my turning on the hot-water tap in my bathtub. As the water ran, I poured in all that was left of a jar of lemon-scented bubbling bath salts. Steaming fragrance filled the room as I undressed and the air became warm, humid, and scented. I sank into the tub and the water buoyed me up. It was like becoming part of a warm lemon meringue pie.

My back unkinked, at first with a little series of aches that turned into sighs as the ghosts of muscular tension whirled away. My knees almost whimpered with delight as they realized they didn't have to support my body. My mind let go too, and I lay stuporous, just conscious enough to add hot water when the bath came near body temperature.

I patted a pile of soapsuds and some bubbles flipped up and sailed into the air. I batted at them and they stuck to my hand. I flicked my fingers and the bubbles flew off in many directions, a mosaic of minuscule rainbows.

I hadn't realized how tense I was. You don't, until you get a chance to relax. And the last two days had been a treadmill.

Worry about McCoo never left my mind. McCoo had saved my life, once in reality and figuratively more than once. I had to save him now, but there didn't seem to be any way to do it. With Shelly Daniello's story so full of holes, he was in trouble. He looked bad, no matter who turned out to have leaked the stories to the press.

And no matter who had bombed McCoo's office and killed Bramble.

This made me feel cold and I added more hot water.

Was the bomber the same person who had been trying to bring McCoo down by leaking to the press items that made the press think he was covering up for Shelly Daniello? A top cop? Would anybody go to such extreme lengths just for the chance—not the certainty—to be superintendent? Cleary?

I thought about Cleary.

Whenever a reporter interviews a person, there's a stepping-back process. If I like the person I'm interviewing, I can't let that liking distract me so much that I don't ask the important questions. I can't be made so fuzzy-cheerful by his charm that I don't ask hard questions. And the opposite holds true, too, of course. Just because I dislike somebody doesn't mean I shouldn't give him a chance. I have to be fair, and nice.

Being nice had been hard in Cleary's case. I didn't take a liking to him. He might be the person who killed Bramble. And if so, he had probably done it while trying to kill McCoo.

If Cleary was the killer, I loathed him.

But I also had to remember that Cleary might not be the killer. McCoo had four possible enemies—five if you counted Superintendent Spurlark. The odds of Cleary's being guilty, therefore, were one in five, or twenty percent. I suppose the chance of his being the killer might be notched up a couple of percentage points because he was first deputy, which maybe put him ahead of the others in the running for superintendent.

When I interviewed Cleary I knew that he was either McCoo's lifetime friend, or possibly a man who wanted to kill him. We're talking deep ambivalence here.

So when I sat down to write the Cleary profile, I had faced a real challenge.

I had no power, only guile. If I wanted to get all the top cops to talk with me, obviously I had to make them *want* to talk with me. The way to do that was to print the first interview right away, the one with Cleary, so the rest of them would be jealous. Unfortunately, the way to make them jealous was to make the interview with Cleary as complimentary as possible. Unfortunately also, I couldn't use the good things he had said about McCoo. They weren't pertinent to the Cleary profile, and, more important, I didn't want to tip my hand as a friend of McCoo's.

This much was obvious. What was less obvious was whether I was going to be able to make myself leave out the things Cleary said that made him look brutish and outdated.

Shouldn't I show him as I saw him? Didn't I have as much obligation to my journalistic integrity as to McCoo?

This question had taken me, oh, maybe two to three seconds to decide, right there in Cleary's office when I told him, okay, he could check out the interview.

Puff up Cleary. Help McCoo. Journalistic integrity could be massaged later.

Promptly at 9 P.M., the police officer had arrived for the copy of my hastily written article. I attached a note:

Dear Deputy Superintendent Cleary,
    As you know, I am on a tight schedule. If I don't hear from you by midnight I will fax the copy to *Chicago Today*.

Thanks,
Cat Marsala

No wonder I had immediately taken a bath.

Ring. The phone. Damn. I was so comfortable here in the hot water. Well, that's what I have a machine for. Let the machine pick up. I could hear the call from the tub; small wonder, since it was only ten feet from here to the phone.

A familiar voice: "Miss Marsala, this is Mr. Whillis. I would like to bring a prospective tenant around to see the apartment tomorrow. If you are not there, I will simply let myself in." Short pause. "Miss Marsala, try to leave the place in decent condition."

Damn. Double-damn! Triple-damn. Unfortunately, he had the right to come in. It was in the contract. I'd looked.

Images flickered through my mind. I could leave some water on the leaky windowsill. Throw clothes all over the floor, demonstrating how piddling tiny the bedroom closet was. Leave several coats on the sofa, demonstrating that there was no coat closet at all. Then wilder visions occurred. Put a piece of rotten meat under a floorboard. Throw a bucket of tea up and stain the ceiling and make it look as though the pipes above leaked.

But I wouldn't. I'm too stupidly well-brought-up. I would put away my clothes and clean the sink and put Long John Silver in his cage. He hates to spend the whole day in his cage. Poor baby.

Oh well, he needs must go whom the devil drives.

And what exactly does that mean, anyway?

This called for the addition of even more hot water.

I'd gotten approximately nowhere so far—or, if anything, worse than nowhere. I'd pretty much confirmed that McCoo was wrong about Shelly Daniello. No facts supported her story.

Well, at least the problem was becoming clearer.

It had two separate aspects, and the one baby step forward I had been able to make was reaching the conclusion that they really were separate.

One of the top cops had been waiting for a break. Waiting, maybe hoping, for a case to come up that potentially could embarrass McCoo. Daniello killing Jurack was perfect.

Up there at the top of the department, one of those people had heard the news, heard of the death of Jurack and the plight of Shelly Daniello—who within hours of the shooting would be facing a round table for the killing—and had thought, This is it. A cop kills a cop, who is a relative. It's got human interest. This is my chance.

Nasty. And very cruel.

Which of them would be that nasty?

Cleary?

I soaped my toes.

Cleary seemed to be McCoo's friend. He had certainly defended McCoo to me, and with no obvious need to. Cleary would not have connected me with McCoo, unless he closely followed the cases McCoo was working on—no, not even then. I had not been involved in cases McCoo was working on, except tangentially and anonymously. Usually I was researching a case of my own and went to McCoo for help.

Could Cleary have realized that McCoo had occasionally cleared up the mess left over from a case of mine? It really didn't seem likely.

McCoo said he and Susanne and the Clearys went to dinner together once a month. Could McCoo have talked about me, just chatting? Something like, "I have this reporter friend, and let me tell you what sort of idiot mess she's gotten herself involved in now."

And if he had, why hadn't he remembered it and warned me?

During the interview I had felt that Cleary was smarter than he looked. Maybe he had been smart enough to know exactly what I was doing the whole time I was in his office. Maybe he had praised McCoo to disarm me.

With that thought, even adding hot water didn't help. I felt chilly and worried.

Then I heard a sound. It was a rustling in the apartment.

You are so vulnerable in a bath.

There was a tap on the floor just outside the door and I leaped up, scattering soapsuds everywhere. I grabbed the toilet brush, ready to defend myself.

Long John Silver hopped in and dropped his rubber toy mouse on the mat.

"Damn! You idiot!" I said, flopping back down in the water. A wave overflowed the edge and splashed him. "Serves you right."

He said, "There is a tide in the affairs of men which taken at the flood leads on to fortune."

"Not in my case, it doesn't."

I threw soapsuds at him and got out of the tub.

By twelve, Cleary hadn't called. He was satisfied with the job of puffery I'd done, as well he should be. I faxed the story to Hal and went to bed.

· 15 ·

"I have a theory about flavored coffees," Harold McCoo said.

"Lay it on me, O Wise One."

"Please!"

"Go on." We were having an early-morning latte in the Loop. And I mean early. It was six-thirty Saturday morning. McCoo wanted to catch up on his work and was willing to work all weekend if necessary. Coffee plus a scone would constitute breakfast for me. McCoo's wife Susanne had already fed him, which didn't stop him from having a scone of his own. We were making a list of whom he needed to approach to pave the way for me. He had said Shelly Daniello's partner, Brad Hubner, ought to be at the top of my list. He'd met Hubner a couple of times, but did not know him well.

Now McCoo stopped sipping and glanced around.

"You go into one of these coffee bars," McCoo said, "it smells great. Or one of these bookstores with the coffee bar in back. Hazelnut coffee, Amaretto coffee, brandied walnut coffee, cinnamon-cognac-nutmeg-filbert-vanilla coffee."

"Mmmm."

"Mmm, yes. But the coffee itself doesn't taste any better. It smells great, but I think the great smell is from some aromatic ingredient, more scent than flavor. The coffee itself isn't so wonderful. And part of the reason probably is that the coffee companies don't use their very finest coffee in brewing flavored coffee."

"Makes sense. Why should they, if the customer is into brandied walnuts rather than coffee?"

"Exactly. Whereas me—I think the proper way to choose coffee is the way you would choose a wine. What kind of bean is it and where was it grown? Then how was it handled after harvest? How was it roasted? That's what you really need to know."

"Smell the hazelnut cream but drink the Kenyan brune?"

"In a word, yes."

"I'm certainly glad you straightened me out on this."

"Listen, I admire Harold McCoo a lot, but I'm telling you right now I'm not gonna lie for him," Brad Hubner said.

"Lie for him?"

"I'm not gonna slant my statement. What I saw is what I saw."

"Has McCoo ever asked you to lie for him?" I was getting angry, and trying hard not to show it.

"No. But I hardly know him."

"Have you ever heard of his asking anybody to lie?"

"No."

"Why do you think he would now?"

"Maybe there was never a good reason before."

"Wait a minute. Do you think he's the sort of person who asks somebody to lie?"

"He's got this great reputation. But like I say, I don't know him very well. And everybody lies if they really get their tit in a wringer, don't they?"

I had caught Hubner, Shelly Daniello's partner, at 7:30 A.M., after the end of an 11 P.M. to 7 A.M. tour of duty, at Sofir's in the Loop, where his cronies in the First District station told me Hubner liked to eat breakfast. Fortunately, he was alone. It wasn't necessary to cut him out of the herd.

Hubner was stocky, maybe thirty-five, just starting to thicken around the middle. The plate of scrambled eggs with four plump sausages, thickly sliced bread with lots of butter, and a side of home fries might explain the waistline. His eyes were pale blue, with very dark eyebrows. His hair was cut nubbin-short, marine-style, showing pale scalp. He jabbed half a sausage and shoved it in his mouth.

I said, "Hey, look, no need to argue." Opening my notebook cover in order to look businesslike and avoid snapping at him, I took a breath. "Tell me what happened that day. And don't slant anything."

"Well, I never wanted a woman for a partner in the first place. Ride around all day, you got a woman partner, there are a lot of things you can't talk about."

"Uh-huh. Such as?"

"Well, you know."

"That's important?"

"You wouldn't ask if you were a guy." He mashed extra butter into his potatoes and shoveled up a big forkful. "Plus," he mumbled over the food in his mouth, "you get into something really bad, they're not going to back you up."

"They won't?"

"Yeah, they don't have the guts."

"Daniello fail to back you up someplace?"

"Well, not yet."

"Ever get into a tight spot, something bad?"

"Yeah. Hey! Waitress!"

"She run away on you?"

"One time we got a shots-fired call, went slidin' in there fast, I'm getting out on my side of the car and she's getting out on hers, and a slug hits the hood of my car. I take off after the shooter, but she comes along like thirty feet behind me."

"Which side of the car was the shooter on?"

"Waitress! Which side? My side." A waitress in a pink apron hurried over. "I need another order of toast, sweetheart. Grape jelly this time."

"So she had to get around to your side to follow you?"

"Yeah, well. Okay. Maybe that's not a great example."

"What kind of a person is she?"

"What kind? I didn't pay all that much attention."

"Oh, come on. Describe her. Some people are talkative, some are quiet. Some are self-righteous, some are adaptable. Some are assertive, some go along with the program. Some are cheerful, some are sour. You know what I mean."

"She was bossy. Irritable. Wanted to do things her way. She certainly wasn't adaptable."

"In what way?"

"Every way."

"Give me an example."

"You know how we get to go to lunch in the middle of our tour. I mean, it's called lunch, no matter what time of day it is, because it's in the middle of our workday, even if it's at night?"

"Yes, I know."

"Well, you're working an eleven-to-seven tour, you're looking for lunch at three A.M. There aren't so many places open. That's why a lot of us eat at the hospital cafeterias."

"Okay."

"Well, Daniello didn't like that. She always wanted to go to this place on Chestnut, Greek cook, open all night."

"And you didn't like that place? What did they make?"

"Basically eggs or pancakes. I like eggs for breakfast. I don't want eggs at three A.M., when I'm in the middle of work. I want a burger or a steak sandwich. Or, like the Northwestern Hospital cafeteria has really fine beef stew."

"I can see why the ambience at the hospital might not be all that relaxing."

"Screw ambience. It's the food that counts."

"So what did you do?"

"Every other tour we had to go to the Greek's."

"In other words, every other night you go to the hospital?"

"Yeah."

"Give and take?"

"Yeah. You couldn't reason with her."

"I see. How long have you been partners?"

"Eighteen months."

"Who have you got now that she's on suspension?"

"A guy named Henry Jackson."

"Does he like the hospital?"

"No. He likes the all-night McDonald's. Which isn't bad. Maybe I won't ever have to take her back, what with all this business."

"Right. So what about this business? What actually happened?"

"Okay. Okay. It was like this. We get this domestic-disturbance call. We go screamin' over there, and does she tell me it's her sister's place? She does not."

"You mean you were already in the house when she told you?" That wasn't what Daniello had said.

"Oh, she told me when we were gettin' out of the car—"

"Really?"

"Or maybe we were still in the car, but shit! Little late, huh? Anyhow, we go running in, and I hear the sister screaming, 'Help! Help! He's gonna kill us!' So Daniello, she just runs in the door. No knock. She's yelling, 'Jurack! You get away from her,' even though she's not in the television room yet. I'm runnin' in, and I get inside the screen door and run smack into the bend in the wall. I was wearing my sunglasses. Broke one of the lenses. Seventy-five-dollar glasses, too. Nearly broke my nose. So I kind of reel back, and I hear the sister, she's still screamin' and yellin', and I hear Daniello bark at the guy, 'Freeze! Police!' Now, I ask you, if you were this guy, you want your sister-in-law to yell 'Police!' at you, like you're some kind of busboy, and when she says jump, you jump?"

"Maybe she wanted him to know it was official. That he was in trouble if he didn't comply."

"Doesn't work if you're a woman. No authority. Works worse if you're a woman relative."

"Maybe it would have worked better if you had been there with her."

He stared at me a few seconds, then threw his head back and said, "You can't help accidents. Anyhow, I got there in half a minute. I'm comin' in right behind her when she shoots."

"Did you see the actual shot fired?" Daniello had said he hadn't.

"No. No, I didn't see the actual shot fired. Don't ask me a hundred times if I did, because I didn't. I don't know how close he was when she fired. Soooooorry! I get there and she's startin' to lean toward Jurack, and the sister's yellin', 'Don't hurt him!' I mean, this woman, one minute it's 'Help me! Help me!' and the next minute it's 'Don't hurt him.' If there's one thing I hate it's these domestic-violence calls. Fuckin' women don't know whether they want him killed or given the Congressional Medal of Honor. Shit. So I run in and there's the knife on the floor, and the guy's crumpling down, and the sister is screamin' bloody murder, and there's this little dumb kid standing there drooling with her hands stuck in her shirt."

"The child was there when you got there?"

"Knew you were gonna ask that. Hey, waitress! Coffee here! Yes. She was there all along. Hadda be. I came in the only door. She was standin' real still against the wall. Couldn'ta got there from the door in the time it took me to come crashin' in. Standin' real still, droolin' away. Shit! Just like her mother. Some people. Whole family of lamebrains, don't have the sense God gave a cucumber."

McCoo came out of his office trailed by three detectives. "Hi, Cat. Be with you in a minute. Fred, I need the lab paper on the Milosevic investigation."

Fred cocked his head. "It's on your desk, boss."

"Great. Tracy, get me the tape again."

"Sure thing."

McCoo told one of the detectives, "Barclay, get back to the ATF and tell them they cooperate with us or else. They know explosives have taggends. They're sitting on something. It can't be taking this long."

"Yes, sir."

"And Jimmie," he said to another, "they have to get final samples. Tell the ME Bramble's funeral is gonna be Tuesday whether he likes it or not."

"But boss, he thinks somebody is gonna ask for more later."

"I know that. Tell him to take everything he needs now. Take extra. I'm not going to keep that family waiting for the body. It's just not right."

"Yes, sir."

"Go with Jimmie," he said to the third detective, who was the size and shape of the Merchandise Mart. "Loom over them."

"Yes, sir."

The detectives left. McCoo said to me, "Found out one thing."

"What was it?"

"The letter bomb was detonated with an air-bag detonator. That's a change of pace."

I looked at Fred, who cocked his head as if to say, "See?"

Russell got up and moved to the file cabinet. The phone rang. Tracy answered. "Yes, he is. Yes sir, I'll tell him."

She hung up with that tight look on her face that people in highly hierarchical organizations get when Somebody High Up calls. "That was Bannister's ADS, boss," she said.

"What did he want?"

"The deputy superintendent wants to see you in his office."

"Now?"

"Now."

McCoo walked out the door without stopping for papers, for a last-minute hair combing, for anything. Bannister was McCoo's long-time mentor, and also what McCoo would call a friend. I had my doubts about that. At any rate, he was McCoo's immediate superior.

Tracy, Fred, Russell, and I hesitated for a few seconds after he left, but there wasn't much to say. Wait and see what was happening. "You're all here, even though it's Saturday?" I asked.

Russell said, "You bet. It's catch-up time."

"I was the only one scheduled," Tracy said. "But we have to reconstruct so much that's missing . . ." She glanced at Bramble's place again.

Russell said, "Cat, there's something we ought to talk about . . ."

Meanwhile, Fred had pulled some CPD lab-report sheets and handed them to me. Fred waited while I studied them. Russell leaned over to look at them too. His ear was freshly bandaged. This bandage was much smaller than the first one, just an ordinary gauze square taped over the ear.

"Okay," I said. "Daniello carried a Model 439 Smith and Wesson nine-millimeter as her side arm of choice. She gave it to the tech people after the shooting, so that it could be tested and matched to the slug in Jurack's body. Am I right so far?"

"Right. Ballistics takes it and fires it into a tank of water. They compare the markings to the round found in Jurack," Fred said. "Look at the next sheet."

I did.

"So this tells us they tried firing her gun at different distances—"

"They use white blotting paper and fire the Smith at zero inches, one inch, two, three, four, five, six, twelve, and twenty-four inches. Then they look at the pattern of burning from the flame, tiny specks of metal, carbon, grease, burned and unburned powder, and stuff like that."

"Don't they already know how far from the gun muzzle a piece of cloth has to be to get burned by the flame? And how far powder shoots out and so forth?"

"Not—"

"I mean, I can see how it would be different for different calibers. A .357 magnum would probably throw metal flecks farther than a .22 target pistol, because it's more powerful. But don't they just have a library of standard burn patterns from standard weapons?"

"Only generally. You get burning from the flame at maybe

AWAITING REPLY FROM			ENTER INTO COMPUTER:		DATE (DAY-MO-YR)
☐ FIELD INQUIRY	☐ COMPUTER	N ☐ (Not In Custody)		Y ☐ (In Custody)	
DIST	BEAT	INQUIRING OFFICER			TIME - INQUIRY

INDIVIDUAL

☐ NCIC ☐ NAME CHECK ☐ TVB	NAME (LAST - FIRST - MI)				
	ADDRESS				

SEX	RACE	DRIVER'S LICENSE NO.		DOB (DAY - MO - YR)	AGE
WGT	HEIGHT	I.R. NO.		SOC. SEC. NO.	

VEHICLE

☐ REGIS. ☐ H & C ☐ NCIC	STATE LICENSE NO.	CITY VEHICLE LICENSE NO.
	VIN	R.D. NO.

REGISTERED TO (NAME)	

ADDRESS	REC?—BEAT OF RECOV.
	☐ YES
	DATE RECOVERED
	☐ NO

ARTICLE

☐ LOCAL ☐ NCIC	TYPE OF PROPERTY
BRAND NAME	R.D. NO.
SERIAL NO.	MODEL NO.

GUN

☑ REG ☐ NCIC	SERIAL NO. 66274-C3	R.D. NO.
MAKE S+W	TYPE OF GUN Model 439	BARREL	CITY REGISTRATION NO. 78743 D
CAL. OR GAUGE 9 m m	INVENTORY NO.	FIREARMS IDENTIFICATION NO.

REMARKS

	☐ SEE OTHER SIDE

LOCAL SEARCH	LEADS SEARCH	NCIC SEARCH
☑ CLEAR ☐ HOT ☐ HOLD	☑ CLEAR ☐ HOT ☐ HOLD	☑ CLEAR ☐ HOT ☐ HOLD

REC'D—OPR NO.	INQ BY—OPR NO.	ANS BY—OPR NO.	APPROVED BY—SUPERVISOR

CPD–31.230-A(4/75)   FIELD INQUIRY, CHICAGO POLICE

zero to two inches. You don't get hardly any particles at more than a foot away. But every gun is a little different. Different types of ammunition fit tighter or looser in a barrel. Looser you get more flame. The length of the barrel makes a difference, too. Plus, ammo isn't all identical, not even the same brand. So they test the actual weapon with the actual ammo. From the same batch, if they can get it."

"I suppose Daniello can't object to their being careful."

"Not except for the results," Fred said grimly.

Ben Jurack had been wearing an undershirt, one of those things with no sleeves and a low neck. The bullet had penetrated the cloth right in the middle of his breastbone, in other words it must have hit the right side of his heart. A good shot, Shelly.

The fabric of the undershirt showed a small amount of scorching. Metal particles were embedded in the fabric. Burned and unburned powder and some gun oil had been detected on the shirt.

This was entirely consistent with the pathologist's report. Dr. Suvitha had said that some of Jurack's chest hairs had been burned, and a few pieces of metal had embedded themselves in his skin, above the point where the undershirt ended. The wound lay behind the cloth of the shirt, and there were fibers from the shirt in the wound. Her opinion was that the muzzle of the weapon had been near Jurack, not at zero inches—no gas in the wound—but possibly between one and seven inches.

The opinion of the lab was pretty similar: four inches away, plus or minus two.

I sighed. "Damn! Absolutely nothing supports Daniello's story."

Fred said, "I know."

"How many rounds in a Smith and Wesson 439?"

"Eight. And the option of one in the chamber."

"And she fired one. You could argue she fired only enough to stop him. If she'd been angry and out of control, she could have fired off all nine."

"Yeah," Fred said. "There's no evidence that she was out of control. But is that good or bad? It certainly doesn't exclude the possibility that she executed him. Still, nobody's said she made any threats. She has a good departmental record—"

He stopped talking because McCoo came in the door.

One glance at McCoo's face and we all knew there was trouble. He stopped inside, closed the door, took a breath and held it. I think the rest of us held our breaths, too.

I felt like saying, "Come on, tell us." But I waited.

McCoo finally said, "He's taking me off the Daniello investigation. He's appointing a task force. We drop it, and we don't touch it again."

· 16 ·

"Drop it?" I said stupidly. "How can you drop it? If you don't get to the bottom of it, you'll—"

My voice tapered off and then stopped dead. He knew what I had been starting to say, though.

"If I don't get to the bottom of it," McCoo finished, "my name is mud."

"Uh, well, yes."

McCoo walked to his office, me trailing after him, Fred, Tracy, and Russell staying behind in a worried group. I said, "Maybe that's what Spurlark and Bannister want."

"Exactly," McCoo said. "If this 'task force' doesn't explain what happened at the Jurack house, Superintendent Spurlark can just demote me, and make it look like I was the problem and I've been taken care of."

"And if they *do* explain what happened at the Jurack house," I said, "then it will look like you weren't able to solve it yourself and they came in and did it for you."

"Yes. Even if they show that I was right, and Daniello's story was right—if they take a little while to accomplish it, nobody will even remember what I said in the first place. And by then it won't help to tell the media 'I told you so.' Their memories are too short."

"Can they *make* you drop it?"

"Of course. What do you think the CPD is, a democracy?"

"No, I guess not. Who's on this task force?"

"Somebody from IAD, a representative from the mayor's office, one of the assistant state's attorneys. And, according to

Bannister, 'three hand-picked investigators from the Detective Division.' "

"Whose hand is picking them?"

"Bannister's, I guess."

"And I imagine they report directly to him?"

"Yep."

"Bannister is supposed to be your friend."

"Yes. Well. He's acting on the instructions of the superintendent. He was very careful to tell me that."

"What gives Bannister the know-how to pick this detective team?"

"Actually it's not that far-fetched, Cat. He was chief of detectives from 1984 to 1988."

"I didn't know that. Or I'd forgotten."

McCoo gazed fixedly at his desk, then at the wall.

"He doesn't sound like a friend, McCoo," I said.

"He was very uncomfortable. And he's not his own boss, Cat. If the superintendent tells him to do something, he has to do it."

"He could resign in protest."

"Well, sure, but that's out of the question."

"Why? He's got his pension locked in. If he's asked to do something he thinks is wrong—"

"This isn't that wrong. It's unfair to me, but it's not as if it's a real moral wrong."

I said, "Okay. Okay. Go ahead; defend the guy. McCoo, what will they investigate? You've *already* investigated."

"I know that. They'll do a cosmetic job. They'll go over what my people and I did. They'll re-interview everybody. They'll find minor discrepancies. People's memories change. Some of the changes, they'll say, 'See, this is important.' But probably it won't be. Or they'll ask some question we didn't ask, like . . . like 'What color shirt was Mrs. Jurack wearing? You said it was dark pink and now you're saying light red.' And then tell the press we didn't ask questions we should have."

"I understand. But, umm, McCoo?"

"What?"

"Don't say that in an interview, if the press asks. I know what you mean and most people would agree with you if they knew the facts, but when you say it, unfortunately, you sound defensive."

He shook his head slowly back and forth. He wasn't telling me he didn't agree. He was shaking his head about the nature of mankind. "I'm not going to be giving any interviews, Cat."

I said, "Now, what does this do to my investigation of Daniello?"

"Kills it."

"McCoo—"

"As far as the department knows, anyway. Officially."

"But I was already unofficial and unknown to them."

"I can't make contacts for you anymore. They could find out. I can't send you back to the medical examiner. I can't put you in touch with the lab people here. You can't do anything that looks official."

"Aha. But I'm still a reporter."

"Exactly. It's a free country. It is outside of this building, anyhow. You can interview anybody who will talk with you as a reporter."

"Can I come here? To your office?"

"Only in emergencies."

"And, of course, when I interview people, I don't mention your name."

"Pretend you never heard of me."

Before I left, McCoo made me a Xerox of the powder stippling and the ballistics report. He told Russell, Fred, and Tracy simply to keep quiet on the Jurack investigation altogether. I was to take my Xeroxes home and leave them there and not tell anybody I had them. Apparently, if I were to use them for liners in the bottom of Long John Silver's birdcage, that would be a good move.

I'd had another, unsettling thought in the depths of last night, a thought that I wanted to run past McCoo. But he wouldn't like it, and I didn't want to hit him with it right now. Life had dumped on him at least once too often, and I couldn't quite assess how well he was holding up. For some reason, I was finding him hard to read today. Was he angry? Sad? Resigned? Depressed? Resolute? Usually I could tell, but not now.

Marie Jurack lived, inappropriately enough, at the corner of Barcourt and Sunnyside Street, northwest of the Loop. In the 1800s there had been a whorehouse not far from here, at Sunnyside and Clark, operated by a three-hundred-pound madam named Gentle Annie. She is said to have run a classy place, chatting with the customers, asking them tony things like "Who's your favorite poet?"

The Jurack apartment was in a four-story U-shaped brick building. There are thousands of these in Chicago, all virtually identical. Maybe somebody in the 1930s had been selling the same building plan cheap all over the city, or maybe this was such a simple structure it could be put up without plans.

The complex contained apartments on four aboveground floors and a half-buried basement floor. There appeared to be eight apartments per floor. The belowground units were now being called "garden apartments." A sign near the door offered one for rent. The lawn in the middle of the U was raked and mowed, but thin. Even at this time of year, when Chicago is mainly brown and gray, there is a difference between a thick brown lawn and a tired brown lawn. This one was tired.

The garden apartments and the first-floor apartments had the extra bonus of back doors that opened onto cement slabs. Upper floors had rear exit doors, presumably for fire-code reasons, but they were up exterior wood stairs that were open to the weather.

A warm breeze whipped dust past the corner of the building. This time of the year, we have a substance I think of as winter's dust. It's what's left of all the pieces of paper, soot, dog droppings, dry leaves, potato chips, pigeon feathers, hot-dog buns, and mittens that have been lying under the snow all winter. Winter's dust made whirlwinds in the warm breeze. The warmth made me uneasy. At this time of year, we often pay for a mild snap with a turbulent, bitter comeuppance.

I was surprised that Shelly Daniello not only had called her sister for me but was willing to go along and introduce me. Maybe she had come to trust me. Or maybe she didn't, and wanted to keep an eye on me. Or maybe she was just plain desperate and hoped something would come of it. I had not told her about McCoo's problem. If she found out and objected to dealing with me now that I was even more unofficial, I'd think of some excuse. But why should she object? She needed as many people on her side as she could get.

We parked on the street, never an easy thing to do in Chicago. "If this wasn't the middle of the day," Shelly said, "you'd never get a place here."

"I believe that."

"Whole lifelong friendships with neighbors have died over parking spaces here. During blizzards, people leave chairs in their parking places when they go to work. If somebody moves the chairs and parks, their cars get sabotaged."

"What do the cops do about that?"

"What can we do? We discourage the practice of leaving chairs out. But how are you gonna trace who's poured sugar in a gas tank? Sugar isn't tagged the way, say, gelignite is."

Marie Daniello Jurack opened her front door. She was taller than the average woman, but not nearly as tall as Shelly, and was not the thoroughbred horse that Shelly was, either. She managed to make tall look short.

Her hair was a middling brown, blunt cut, and largely ignored by its owner. The part was straight, but the style was nil. She wore a brown skirt that was clean but hung down farther on one side than the other, awkward brown flat-heeled shoes, and a tan knit shirt. There was a fresh scar with stitches still in place visible along her jawline.

I said, "How do you do, Mrs. Jurack?"

"Okay," she said, and turned to lead us into the room.

She showed no curiosity. Now, I'm aware that life can be hard. I'm aware that the nature of chance is such that some people have more bad luck than others. Certainly people do get beaten down. But people who have no curiosity in their eyes, who show no interest in anything, who find nothing surprising about life, let alone amusing—people like that scare me.

Shelly said, "Cat would like to look around."

"You told me," Marie responded, still walking toward the kitchen. She didn't even glance back over her shoulder.

"And then chat with you a little bit."

Marie Jurack turned briefly at this remark.

"Why?" she said.

After a two-second beat, Shelly said, "Why not?" And this seemed to be response enough for Marie Jurack.

We crossed a living room in which a brown sofa and a beige-and-brown plaid chair shouldered up to a corner table with a couple of small framed photos on it. In front of the sofa and chair was a glass-topped table with a base made of sil-vered elephants. There was a curio cabinet with figurines. There was not a speck of dust visible. There also was not a book or even a magazine in sight. The carpet looked like oat-meal and the ceiling was the texture of cottage cheese.

The kitchen was mainly pink, pink walls and a gray-and-pink floor. It was bigger than mine, but all kitchens are bigger than mine. A white stove faced a green refrigerator. Both were clean. The floor was clean. A dinette made of steel legs and a pink-and-gray plastic top was clean too. There was no fruit out on the counter. There was no cookie jar. There were no herb plants on the windowsill. There were no plants, period. There was just one homey touch. On the floor was a cat litter box and it was scrupulously clean, too, raked like a Japanese garden. Still, I was encouraged to see it.

Marie led us toward a door off the kitchen. "This is where it happened," she said. She was pointing into a small room, rather dim, with a television set at the far end. It was on. The voice of Edward Everett Horton chuckled from the speakers.

The shades were half lowered on the window. The whole room was no more than twelve by twelve feet. I looked down at the floor, which was bare wood.

"I got rid of the rug," Marie Jurack said pointedly.

An old green sofa and two old chairs faced the television. This was the sort of room where you put furniture too good to throw out but too dilapidated for display in the front room. In the middle of the sofa sat a little girl wearing blue bib overalls.

"This is Belinda," Shelly said. Here was the child they called Beanbag.

The little girl was watching a rerun of "Rocky and Bullwinkle," a particular favorite of mine. "Oh, the metal-munching moon-mice episode! I wish I could watch this," I said, earning a smile from Beanbag and a skeptical glance from Shelly. But I was serious. I love that show.

The door we stood in was the only entrance to the room. Because of its small size, Jurack could not have been very far away from Daniello when she shot him, even if she was just barely inside the door.

Jurack had fallen, they said, with his feet close to the television set and his head near the sofa; in other words, his head had been nearer to the door. "Shelly, where exactly did he lie after he fell?" I whispered this to her, because I didn't want to make Beanbag's memories any worse.

Daniello whispered back, "About here," and put her toe on a spot about a yard from the doorway.

"And where were you?" I whispered.

"About where I am now." She was just inside the door, less than eighteen inches from Jurack's head.

"Had you stepped back as he fell?"

"Maybe a little."

I sighed. It was all possible. Unfortunately, it was possible either way.

And what about Beanbag being there at the time of the shooting? Brad Hubner had seen Beanbag standing against the wall near the corner at the far end of the sofa. I looked. That placed her at the far corner from the door. The child must have been in the room all along.

And what about the bruise on Jurack's head? The sofa and the chairs were the overstuffed variety, with no exposed wood anyplace. No coffee table. No wastebasket. No sharp edges. The TV set was too high to fall on, and besides, he fell away from it, toward Daniello. I saw no object whatever that he could have fallen against to make that bruise on the side of his head. This was definitely a second black mark against Daniello's story.

For a minute I studied the room, but it didn't reveal anything else.

Shelly Daniello took charge. Just as well, since her sister wouldn't and I probably shouldn't. Cops learn to take charge.

"Let's go talk in the living room," she said.

She got me ensconced on the beige plaid chair and her sister on the sofa. "Now, I'm going to run to the corner and get us all a cappuccino mocha. I'll be right back."

She was doing this on purpose, of course, to give me time alone with Marie, even though her sister showed no awareness. I figured I had better use the time that Shelly had given me.

"Mrs. Jurack, can I ask you some questions?"

"I don't see why not. Everybody else has."

"Well, I don't want to be too aggress——to offend you. I mean, with your husband recently dead . . ."

I waited but she said nothing at all. And it had not really been a question.

"Was Belinda in the room when the shooting took place?"

"I took her out of the room, after."

"But was she there before? Before it started?"

"Um. The television was on."

"But did you actually *see* her in there?"

"I don't remember. I was kind of upset." She was being hit by Jurack, of course.

"Well, after Shelly arrived, did you see Belinda come in the room?"

"I was kind of too upset."

I sighed. She seemed to have no interest in the questions. Didn't she care about her sister's trouble? On the other hand, maybe it was a good thing that I didn't sense her trying to protect Daniello. If she tried to invent facts to help Shelly, it might be endearing, but it would only make figuring out what really happened all that much more difficult. "Mrs. Jurack, it's generally believed that Mr. Jurack had a long history of spousal abuse."

"Yes."

"Well, how did you feel about that?"

"He shouldn't've hit me."

"What did you do to stop him?"

"I asked him to stop. A couple of times I reported him to the police."

"What happened?"

"Nothing much. His buddies came around."

"And did what?"

"Told him to stop. One of them laughed, but most of them told him to stop."

"Did that make him stop? For a while?"

"Not very long," she said flatly.

"Mrs. Jurack, that must have been horrible for you."

"Yeah. It was."

"And for Belinda."

"Yes."

Would this woman *never* show emotion? I was getting frustrated. All right, I'd forget her problems, and concentrate on Daniello's problems.

"Was Jurack attacking Shelly when she shot him?"

"Yeah."

"How far away was he?"

"I don't know. I don't remember. I'm not good at distances."

"If we went into the television room, could you show me where he was?"

"They already asked me to do that. I couldn't remember. Anyway, they were moving. And I was upset at the time."

"Oh. Who asked you?"

"Detectives, I think."

"Mrs. Jurack, are you relieved that he's gone?"

"No, I don't know what I'm going to do now."

"Are you glad Shelly shot him?"

"No. I never wanted her to shoot him."

"But you were screaming for help."

"I was? Well, I sort of was, I guess. I wanted him to stop."

"Stop what?" I knew what, but I wanted to force her to tell me, to verbalize it and confront it.

"To, you know, to stop hitting me."

"Hitting you?"

"Well . . . he . . . this time, he kind of threatened me, too."

"What do you exactly mean by 'threatened'?"

"Oh, with a knife."

"Threatened you with a knife?"

"Yes."

"Just threatened?"

She didn't answer.

"Mrs. Jurack, Marie, you were taken to the hospital, and at the hospital the doctors sewed up three different knife wounds. One on your forearm. That wasn't too bad. It required thirteen stitches, but it was a fairly superficial cut. One on your shoulder. That only took five stitches, because it wasn't wide, but they said it was very deep. It was a stab wound and it was a good thing it was in your upper shoulder instead of farther down your chest, in your lung."

She just stared at me.

"Then there was the wound on your jaw. It slashed from the side of your neck up across the jawline. He was going for your throat. And if you hadn't ducked sideways, he might have cut your throat."

She still didn't say anything, but her right hand went to her neck and her fingertips played along the tiny stitches that tracked her neck like asterisks all in a row.

"And if he had," I said brutally, "he'd have killed you."

She put her right hand in her lap, where it immediately took hold of her other hand and squeezed, appearing to hold the left hand back from making some gesture. In a soft voice that also was without gesture, she said, "He really didn't mean it."

"Well, how much damage would he have done if he *had* meant it?"

She recoiled. Immediately, I felt guilty, as if I, too, had been beating her.

"I'm sorry, Mrs. Jurack. I'm just frustrated that you'd let him bul——I mean, I don't like to see one person hurt another."

"You started to say you're frustrated that I'd let him bully me." She allowed herself a one-sided smile. "You're just like Shelly." I started to ask how she had responded to Shelly in that case, but she said, "You're just like Shelley. You don't understand."

"Then help me understand." She shook her head as if it was impossible. "Tell me about what happened that afternoon, please."

"Well, Ben had come home from work kinda simmering already. I mean, I don't know what had bothered him, exactly, but he was getting that way more and more."

"Annoyed by the job."

"Yeah. That's about right."

"Then what happened?"

"He started yelling at me. I could see it building up. I could always see it starting. He wanted to get a fresh shirt and go out to the neighborhood bar, one he likes called EstaLoca. So he looked in his drawer for a fresh shirt. He pulled his outer shirt off and started throwing shirts out of the drawers."

"And?"

"Well, it was Friday. He wanted a white shirt. Monday is my wash day. Tuesday is my ironing day. There was only blue shirts left."

"You don't buy no-iron shirts?"

"Ben wouldn't wear them. He said they felt slimy."

"Oh. Great. Then what?"

"He got mad. I told him we always do it this way, but he didn't care. He wanted a fresh white shirt. So I said I'd iron him one, but he wanted it right then."

"And naturally—"

"I said I'd hurry, but he was mad by then and he slapped me. Just a small slap."

"Sure. So then what?"

"Well, I . . . it's a funny thing. If you kept him happy, if I kept him happy, he most of the time wouldn't hit me. But it was weird. Almost always, once he started hitting me, it got worse."

"Uh-huh."

"And then, once he starts, you might as well get it over with."

I waited but she didn't go on. "So you two were where at this point? In the living room here?"

"No, in the kitchen. He punched me more, and I said I'd call the police, but he said he didn't believe it, so I grabbed the phone. There's a wall phone in the kitchen, you know? So he grabbed up the knife and cut the phone cord. I'd already called part of 911."

"Would you have gone through with it if he hadn't cut the phone cord?"

She looked at me with a world of hurt in her eyes. I was

sorry I'd asked, but that look probably meant no. "What happened then?"

"It was just sort of bad luck that he had the knife, I guess. He was really mad then. I was yelling, I guess, and he stuck me with the knife and I screamed. I ran around the kitchen and tried to get out of his way, and then I ran into the television room. Real soon after that, Shelly came in."

"So how long did the, uh, fight in the kitchen take?" I didn't want to call it a fight, but I figured she'd prefer that to "torture."

"I don't know."

"Guess."

"It seemed like forever. It seemed like an hour. But I guess it was maybe twenty minutes."

"So Shelley came in—"

"Yeah. I was glad to see her, but I was worried, too. I mean, I knew how she felt about Ben."

"How?"

"She didn't like him."

"Mrs. Jurack, did Shelly shoot your husband intentionally, not really needing to?"

"No!"

"Did she walk up to him, crack him on the side of the head with her gun, stunning him, and then fire point-blank into his chest while he was standing there in front of her?"

She stared at me with her mouth hanging open.

"Did she, Mrs. Jurack?"

"No!"

"Then how did Jurack get that bruise on his head?"

"I don't know. I don't know!"

"Maybe she shot him first, point-blank, right there in front of you. Then he didn't go down fast enough to suit her, so she clipped him on the head with her gun. And then he went down."

"No. No, he was a little bit away from her when she fired. I don't know how far, but not right near."

"Then how did he get the bruise on his head?"

"She never hit him! She never did. I'm telling the truth. She didn't."

"Then how did it get there?"

"I don't know! Please, I'm telling you, I don't know."

But she did know. I was sure of it.

• 17 •

"You know what strikes me about you and your sister—"

"You think we're so different."

"Well, yes." Daniello was smart, and despite being prickly, she was alert to people's feelings. She had brought coffee back to the house, and a hot fudge sundae with peppermint ice cream for Beanbag. We'd had a nice, vague social chat, and Beanbag, a serious little child, had laughed at some of Daniello's jokes, and after thirty minutes of observation I had the feeling that nothing in that family was going to improve unless some major event happened. The abuser was gone, so there wouldn't be any hitting, but Marie's personality was just the same as if he'd been there. It was as if she was still cowering, just in case he walked in.

Finally we left, in my car. I said, "Your sister apparently went on and on, year after year, taking a beating, threatening to leave but never walking out. Like a lot of women, I find it almost impossible to picture myself doing that. I mean, people talk about low self-esteem, but when you're actually being hurt—and I don't mean just hurt, I mean *injured*—don't you run?"

"Humans are pack animals. We need our tribe. We want to be liked and approved of by the people around us. Jurack was her alpha animal."

"That's all very well, but she could have found other people around her to approve of her. You, for example."

"My approval didn't matter much, because I was her sister and therefore always attached to her in some way. She wouldn't lose me no matter what. And because I was a woman. Women's approval doesn't mean as much, either. When Jurack told her she wasn't any good, that mattered to her."

"Did you and Marie grow up in different households?"

"No. Same time, same place. My father was an Old World Italian. Lived on Taylor Street until he made enough money to move north. In our house, my mother did the cringing and my father did the hitting. Traditional family values. When he'd been drinking he'd come home and he'd take out all his frustrations on my mother and us. He was a slapper, not a puncher, really. And a belittler. Tell us we were nothing, how we'd never be anything, how we couldn't even learn to make his coffee right, how my mother never learned to clean the house right. We were stupid. We'd never grow up to be worth anything."

"He did this to both of you?"

"Oh, yeah. One thing you gotta say about my father, he never played favorites."

"So how come you're strong-minded and so—" The word I was looking for was "aggressive," but I didn't want to say it. She knew what I meant, though.

"Pressure. Give you an example. You know how it is when a parent is constantly after a child to eat? 'Finish your dinner' and 'Clean your plate' and 'If you eat all your vegetables you can have dessert.' The kind of parent who forces food on the child?"

"My oldest brother's wife."

"Well, the child will do one of two things. Give in and eat everything and equate food with love, and get fat. Or be disgusted at eating more than she wants and start becoming a picky eater, and get thin."

"That's true."

"That's how pressure works. It distorts. But you can't really tell who will be distorted which way. Well, that was how it was with my father and us. He succeeded in convincing Marie that she was in the wrong and always would be, and he convinced me that *he* was in the wrong and I was right."

*   *   *

"It's so frustrating," I said when I let her out at her apartment building. "You want to scream at her, '*Why do you stand for this?*' But you know it won't do any good."

"Actually, I did scream at her. That very thing. A lot of times. And it didn't do any good."

"I suppose she can't help it."

Shelly said, "Suppose we say Marie was damaged by her upbringing, and it made her subservient even to the point of allowing her child to be exposed to violence. Therefore do we have to sympathize with her?"

"Yeah, I think we do."

"Then can we also say that Ben Jurack had been led by his upbringing to believe he had to punish to be strong? He sure as hell believed that any back talk from his wife meant he was less of a man."

"I suppose he did."

"His father is just like him. So can't we pardon him in the same way we pardon Marie?"

"You're overlooking the fact that he did a wrong thing. Actually, he did a criminal thing. He's a batterer. She's a victim."

"Listen, I'm not saying this is right, I'm just asking. And if Marie was putting Beanbag in danger, how do we justify that?"

I said, "*Jurack* was putting Beanbag in danger."

"Suppose Beanbag was at the beach with Marie. Beanbag gets her foot caught between two rocks. The tide is coming in. Neither the tide nor the rocks are Marie's fault. Doesn't she still have a moral responsibility to get Beanbag out of there?"

"Lord! I suppose."

"Also, Jurack lost the chance to have any real, human relationship with his wife and child. Shouldn't we feel sorry for him?"

"I don't think so."

"Hell, neither do I. But it's worth asking."

I sighed, she sighed, then I sighed again. There were no easy answers.

I said, "Yeah, poor Marie—I mean, 'Get a life' doesn't begin to cover it."

"Exactly."

"So what does your sister do?"

"What do you mean?"

"The background of her life was that her husband beat her. She thinks that's normal, one of the elements of life she can't change. So maybe she goes about her work to make herself forget. What work?"

"Oh. She washes the countertops. And then the floor. Then the bathroom bowl and the kitchen walls. Then the counter-tops again."

I had failed to discover anything that improved Daniello's chances from her sister; in fact, I had confirmed the worst. I had failed to get anywhere with Daniello's partner, Brad Hubner. And the expanded round table would convene Mon-day. There was a distinct possibility that things would get worse for McCoo. If so, I had to level with him about a worry that kept nagging at me. He wouldn't like it. But it would only make things worse for him to be living in a dreamworld.

First, I called Louise Montoya and set up an appointment.

Then I called McCoo. We met at an ice cream parlor on LaSalle for a late-afternoon treat, or consolation food, depend-ing on how you think of it. For me, like Beanbag, hot fudge sauce does a lot of consoling.

"McCoo, tell me this. Do any of the top cops open their own mail?"

"No. They've all got secretaries. Or their ADS."

"Now, at your level—the people like commander of per-sonnel, chief of detectives, that level—do any of those people open their own mail?"

"No."

"So any of the top cops would know that you wouldn't open your mail; Bramble would?"

"Yes."

"And anybody in the organization, anybody in management at least, would have known this."

"Yes."

"And I can tell you that anybody outside the organization would assume a person in your position would have a secretary."

"I know what you're getting at."

"Exactly. There's virtually no chance that the bomb was intended for you. It was intended for Bramble."

He was silent for half a minute. He finally said, "Yes. I've been thinking that, too. When I first realized she might have been the actual target, I wondered if I was trying to make myself feel better."

"In what way?"

"I had been feeling so guilty. That she was killed in my place. It was like I was responsible, in a sense. Like she took the bullet for me."

"I can understand that."

"So I figured I was trying to make myself feel better. But in fact, it would take a pretty stupid assassin to think I'd necessarily open that mail."

"Exactly."

"She could have been a random target."

"With your name on the envelope? I doubt it."

"I suppose not."

"Could Bramble have been targeted because she saw somebody come into your office and take evidence in the Daniello case?"

"And didn't tell me? Never."

"If it was somebody you liked—"

"Not once things got really bad in the press. She wouldn't protect anybody that much."

"Let me ask you something. I'll tie this up, believe it or not. McCoo, I don't think any of the deputy superintendents would have gone into your office and rummaged around. What if they'd been caught?"

"They could bluff it out easier than anybody else could."

"How? How could they explain not having asked you directly for the information?"

"Maybe they needed it in a hurry. Or could claim they did. Whatever."

"No. 'Whatever' doesn't really work, McCoo. Let's be specific. Say some deputy superintendent—say Montoya—wants the autopsy report to see what goodies she can leak to the press and make you look bad. Say the bruise on Jurack's forehead was the info that she eventually leaked. But she doesn't know ahead of time exactly what she's going to find. And she doesn't know your filing system. She's going to come into your office and rummage around in the files and finally maybe locate and pull the autopsy protocol. Now you or Bramble walks in. How's she going to explain why she's there? It's an emergency? What emergency? Her divisions are Training, R and D, Personnel, and Finance. She's gonna claim she's doing an emergency personnel survey and needs to know about all the bruises in the Chicago Police Department?"

"Don't get funny, this is serious."

"And why would she need to know anything, anyway? The Daniello scandal wasn't her problem."

"So okay, so Montoya couldn't make up a good reason."

"All right. But if it was one of the others, it doesn't work, either. The deputies with a genuine need to know should simply have asked you. Cleary, for example. He's first dep. He could just tell his ADS to go and ask you for information. I realize that if he's the leak, he would want *not to have known* it, so that no one would think he *could* leak it, so therefore he couldn't send his ADS, but then we're back where we started. If somebody comes in and finds Cleary or his ADS rummaging in the files, they'll wonder why. In fact, they'll know something's rotten because *he should have told you he wanted it, and then sent his ADS.*"

"True."

"Even if they snuck in at night. Any time of day or night you could be called in on an emergency."

"I—all right, Cat. That's true."

"McCoo. Don't you know what I'm getting at?"

"What?"

"Why not face it?"

He turned away from me. Talk about body language; he truly did not want to face it. I didn't want to either, but somebody had to be hardheaded. And McCoo was too smart not to have thought of it.

"McCoo, none of the deputy superintendents, or the superintendent, would have walked into your office and searched your files. At any time. Not even if they had a key. It would be too risky. They had a confederate."

He didn't say anything.

"Don't tell me it hasn't occurred to you."

He still didn't say anything.

"McCoo. A confederate *in your office.*"

Now he turned back toward me. His face was without expression.

"And the most likely person—"

"No," he said.

"The most likely person was Bramble."

· 18 ·

"No! Not Bramble!"

His hand balled into a fist. He wanted to pound the table, but it was a little round marble thing on wire legs, and in a public place besides.

"Damn! Cat, that's absolutely crazy! How long have you been thinking this stuff?"

"Don't attack me! Tell me why it's wrong."

"Bramble was the most loyal person I've ever known."

"McCoo, I didn't know her nearly as well as you did, but I liked her a lot. I don't want her to have done it. Still, you have to face facts. We don't know what problems she may have had. What personal problems or what financial problems. We know she had a son; maybe he needed money badly. Maybe the top cop promised her money. We don't know what her dreams were. Or her resentments. Maybe he promised her a promotion. One thing I've learned about life is that you can never be sure what another person is thinking."

"Not Bramble."

"Not Bramble? Yes, Bramble. It's true of everybody. Haven't you ever had some longtime friend tell you that he's carried a resentment for years about some minor event that you didn't interpret at all the way he did? It's happened to nearly everybody."

"Well, sure."

"You can*not* know what Bramble was thinking. Maybe she fooled herself that giving a top cop inside information was okay. He had the authority to get the information directly if he wanted. Or she might say to herself it was just a leak, after all. A transmission of data. She didn't alter the evidence. She didn't lie to make you look bad. Perfectly accurate, legitimate information just got out a little early, she might say. There was nothing really *wrong* about it."

"Not Bramble. She wouldn't fool herself like that. Or hurt me, either."

"If not Bramble, it could be Russell, or Tracy, or Fred."

"They're just as loyal as Bramble."

"And less likely. If I read your office accurately, Tracy and Russell and Fred have certain areas they specialize in. Tracy does tapes and 911 records and a lot of the electro-tech stuff. Russell concentrates on personnel. And Fred does most of the medical examiner, lab, ballistic stuff."

"They all fill in for each other."

"Oh, I realize that. I know they all have days off, which means they'd have to be able to do each other's jobs at times. But when they're all there, it would look odd for Fred, for instance, to pull out and listen to court tapes instead of Tracy. Or for Tracy to be searching for information in the personnel files instead of Russell."

"That's true."

"And you told me yourself you weren't showing the Daniello documents around, even in your office, even to Fred, Tracy, and Russell."

"That's true, too."

"Although, they told me they each take a Saturday or Sunday on rotation. They'd be there alone then."

"Right."

"Did the three major leaks appear in the press on a Sunday or Monday?"

"Let me think." He dropped his head on his fist for a few seconds. "One, at most. I think the leak about the child being in the room may have come out on a Monday."

"Not all, though?"

"No, not all."

"See, that confirms what I'm saying. No matter how you look at it, Bramble is the most likely of the four of them. She could have done it anytime. She had easiest access to everything. But there's another piece of evidence that points to her."

"What?"

"She was *killed*, McCoo. That's what I've been getting at. Suppose the top cop covered his traces by shutting her up?"

Our ice cream didn't seem quite so tasty anymore. We went back to McCoo's office. We stood looking at his office safe. Getting a chance to study the papers that had been on Bramble's desk seemed reason enough for me to go back there, but we went separately, and I waited outside one of the courtrooms until the hallway was clear and then slipped in the door.

"We need to find out whether Bramble left any suspicious communications. Like notes from Montoya, Winter, Cleary, or Bannister, for example."

"Damn," McCoo said.

"Or checks."

"I'll have one of the detectives look into her bank account," McCoo said. "If I can't do the Jurack case, at least I can investigate Bramble."

He worked the combination of his small safe. When the door swung open, the smell of smoke seeped out at us. I held my breath a second or two, horrified at how vividly the scent brought back the scene. McCoo sighed from way down in his chest. Unaware he did it, he fingered the side of his head, where he had been struck by the bomb blast.

"Did you go over these?" I asked him.

"No. ATF and Bomb and Arson had been through everything for evidence by the time I got back. You remember. You were here. They'd left it all piled in a corner and locked the office door."

"And you had to send out for the key. And then you and I put the papers in your safe."

"Right. And I've kept the door key since then."

"Anybody else have the combination?"

"No. I don't use the safe for current papers. Just special items. When I was going to be away on vacation I'd leave the key with Bramble."

"All right. So, Bomb and Arson may have taken some papers, but whatever they didn't take should still be here?"

"Absolutely."

Some of the papers were still damp. The edges of some were burned. Some looked as if nothing had happened to them. Because he seemed to be hanging back, I asked, "You want to take half?"

"Sure. Hand me a bunch."

We sat quietly for fifteen or twenty minutes, reading, shuffling papers. It took great care to separate the damp ones without tearing them. We wanted to keep everything as intact as possible. Some of the really soaked, fragile papers I laid out on the windowsill to dry. McCoo found several sheets of office schedules in Bramble's handwriting. "She always managed to be fair to everybody," he said. "People prefer Saturday off, so she was careful to spread the duty around."

"I'm sure."

"There's nothing that looks susp——"

I said, "Hey!"

He snapped, "What?" McCoo was tenser than I had thought. He sat up straight and stared at me.

"Well, I don't know. Don't look so eager. It's just that you never told me there was a follow-up to the autopsy report. I could have asked Dr. Suvitha about it, if I had known."

"There wasn't any."

"Yes, there was. It's right here."

The sheet was headed SUPPLEMENTARY REPORT.

It was dated March 14, but reported on blood drawn the day Jurack was shot.

POSTMORTEM REPORT   DEPARTMENT OF HEALTH   CASE NO.   PAGE
                                    COOK COUNTY   723-96   1 of 1
                                  2121 W. HARRISON
                                  CHICAGO IL 60612

SUPPLEMENTARY REPORT

3-14-97

Subject Off. Shelly M. Daniello.
Sample drawn 3-7-97 at 0420 hours.
Toxicology screen ethanol only as per instructions.
Ethyl alcohol 0.11%

[signature], M.D.

[ALL PAGES MUST BE SIGNED]

MK-050-C

"What the *hell?*" McCoo said.

"Blood alcohol point eleven?"

"You can't legally drive at point eleven!"

"McCoo, do you realize what this means? Shelley Daniello was legally drunk when she shot Jurack!"

"No, it doesn't."

"Why not?"

"It's not right. The medical examiner doesn't draw blood from live people. They do cadavers, period. If Daniello had been tested at all, the blood would have been drawn by the medical tech here and sent to our lab in this building."

"What are you saying?"

"This document is a forgery."

"Really?"

I looked closely at it. I said, "What can we deduce about it? It's not folded. It probably didn't come by mail."

I turned it over and saw the indentations of typewriter keys, filling in blanks on a form set. "It's original, not a fax or a copy. Maybe it was about to be planted in her file."

"That's not the only thing. Wait a minute."

McCoo rummaged around in his papers. He found the Xerox of the medical examiner's autopsy protocol. "Look at Suvitha's signature," he said.

"Oh, wow. They're totally different."

• 19 •

Unfortunately, this bizarre development didn't tell us anything more about who was behind the attacks on McCoo. In fact, it stupefied me. I couldn't think how it fit in. Could Bramble have been planning to discredit Shelly Daniello?

Looking like a man who had been hit with a two-by-four, McCoo locked all the papers back in the safe.

"Now that I think of it, Hubner would have told us if Daniello was drunk," McCoo said.

"Yeah. Gleefully."

I had an appointment with Montoya, and McCoo was too stunned to go on with any serious discussion, or to continue searching the other papers right now, so I left.

On the way to the appointment, I went trolling for more top cops. Gregory Dennison Winter's little bird lady—hard at work on a Saturday afternoon—still believed that Winter was much too busy to talk with a reporter "at this particular time." She implied that the present crisis was responsible. I glanced in his office. He was not reading the paper; he was talking on the phone, saying ". . . whereas, unlike the others, I have done exactly that." You have to wonder whom he would talk to in that stilted way. "Whereas," indeed!

I had no way to know whether he had seen the article I wrote on Bob Cleary.

I entered the superintendent's office. His secretary said, "No, I'm sorry, but he couldn't possibly see you now. Try back in seven days."

Oh, sure. In a week, he might not even be superintendent. On to Louise Montoya's office.

Preconceptions are so stupid. She was an absolutely striking woman, with a thin streak of white in jet-black hair, like a spotlight advertising her high cheekbones. She had piercing dark eyes and thick eyelashes. I had expected a tough, female version of Bob Cleary, with Hispanic coloring. I should have known better, but, of course, I had thought "lifetime Chicago cop." Surely I am too old to be making these mistakes.

"I saw your article on Bob Cleary this morning," she said. Her eyes had a slight crinkle that told me she realized the piece was a puff job. She added, "Very nice. I imagine he liked it."

"I don't know. He hasn't said." After a second or two of reflection, I added, "I'm doing profiles. Not psychoanalyses."

"Mmm-mm. Evidently. So what can I do for you?"

"The same. I'd like to write a profile on you."

"Okay."

"Tell me about yourself."

"Starting where?"

"Wherever you want. It's the same format. A kind of personal sketch. Which doesn't mean it needs to be the same content. My idea is to answer the question 'Who are these people?' "

"I'd like to see what you've written before you publish it."

"Sure." I told her my arrangement with Cleary. She had a fax at home, unlike Cleary, and I promised to send her the final copy. I showed her my tape recorder. "Good," she said. "I'd rather be responsible for my words than yours."

"So why did you want to be a police officer?" I asked.

"I was a neglected kid. I ran with some boys and girls who were out of control and on their way to jail if they didn't straighten up. Some did. Some didn't. One day I watched one of our guys in a fight with another guy. Our guy got hit with a bicycle chain. They don't sound dangerous, compared to a Glock or Tec-9, but when you get hit with a chain and it gets pulled back away from you, it rips off long shreds of skin. I watched, and I knew then that this kid, a handsome guy, maybe nineteen, was going to be scarred for life, right across his face, from his temple down over the edge of his nose and his upper lip. I thought, What's he doing here? and then I thought, What am I doing here? It was like an epiphany. I thought, My life is wasting away here, when someplace else maybe I could make a difference."

I couldn't help saying, "That's very high-minded."

"You're skeptical? Sure, I had other motives. Do human beings ever do anything for one single, pure motive? I was a girl in a culture that thought the men were everything. I had never, never once in my entire life been able to tell a man what to do and he did it. And all my life men had been giving me orders. My father. Grandfather. Brother. All my boyfriends. All my *uncles,* for God's sake. Yeah, I wanted the gun and the badge."

"Did it work out the way you hoped?"

"Not exactly. I came on in 1965. At that point it had been just ten years that women officers were even allowed to wear a uniform. We had these dumb light blue blouses and the regulation shoes were dark blue with a three-inch heel. Skirts and high heels! Guess how well we could run after your basic fleeing felon in that."

"Not very well."

"Right. And then we got criticized for not being as fast on our feet chasing down crooks! 'Girls can't run!' We had to carry the gun in our purses. There was a little clip in there to hold it. Wouldn't be ladylike to wear a gun belt. If somebody attacked us, we had to open the purse and go grabbing around for a weapon. We could've been shot a dozen times over before we got a weapon out. They'd rather have us look ladylike than be safe. We weren't allowed to go out on patrol until 1974."

"I didn't know it was that recent."

"People forget. When the first group of women was being trained for patrol in squad cars, the brass ordered an instructor from a local charm school to come and teach us how to get into and out of a car in a ladylike manner while wearing a skirt."

"I haven't figured that out yet."

"When we were finally allowed in the cars, one of the papers printed a cartoon of a squad car with little ruffled curtains around the windows."

"Did the male officers accept you?"

"Please! Don't ask! No, to be fair, some did. In any group, there are always some grown-ups."

"And some not."

"First day I came on patrol, you know, they didn't have a women's locker room. Why would they, with no women? And of course the men got dressed in the men's locker room. So what the bosses did, this particular district, was they put a set of metal lockers facing the door. At right angles to the other lockers and facing away from them. The other lockers ran along the walls, you see what I mean?"

"Yes. With the doors of your set of lockers facing the front door? So they couldn't see you?"

"Close. So I couldn't see them. I was supposed to go in, get whatever I wanted from my locker, then go to the ladies' bathroom, get dressed there, then go back and put whatever I'd taken off in my locker."

"Wonderful," I said grimly.

"But wait; that's not the whole story. So I go in, my first day, I'm a little bit intimidated, but full of beans too, you know, I'm gonna knock this job. And I go to my locker to get geared up. Open the door and I was *absolutely showered* with Tampax. Little things rolling all over the floor, *ploppeta-ploppeta.*"

"Oh, my Lord. What a mean thing—"

"Well, yeah, it was. But I figured this was it. If I didn't stake out my spot now, I never would. So I jump around the end of the locker, and they're all waiting and quiet, maybe snickering a little bit. And I say, 'Hey, guys! This is really generous! Know how much these little suckers cost?' So, they're all staring. And I say, 'You probably saved me a week's pay here. Listen, anybody got a bag?' "

I was laughing by now.

"So somebody actually had a plastic bag from the laundry or whatever. And I bundled them all into the bag. I asked a couple of the guys to pick up the ones that had rolled into the men's end of the locker room. And they did. All sheepish, and now they're holding them by two fingers. Suddenly they're embarrassed to touch them. I mean, it was one of the funniest things you'll ever see."

I was laughing harder.

"Maybe three years later," she said, "I was partnered with one of those guys. Different district, the Fourteenth. And I asked him something I'd always wanted to know. 'How did you get all those things into the locker?' 'Cause a locker, the door is vertical, and the whole thing was just full, all the way to the top. You can't pile 'em up, because they'll roll. And he said they held a real stiff sheet of paper, four feet long, up against the open locker with just enough room at the top to pour the things in. Then they closed the locker door and pulled the paper out. I said, 'That was very creative.' "

"What did he say?"

"He said he felt guilty about it later. Now don't put that story in the article."

"No. Okay, I won't. You know, not everybody would be able to take something like that in stride."

"Oh, hell, no. I've seen women quit over stuff like that."

"Do you feel that quitting is wimpish of them?"

"No, I really don't. It's not fair to say that a person is a wimp not to like working in a hostile environment. Or that you're a wimp if you don't want to work with people who don't want you. Women today coming on don't realize how bad it was. They aren't aware of the gains we've made."

"How do you explain the way you've risen to the top?"

"Single-mindedness. I love my work. I'm married. My husband and I have no children. He's a sports therapist. We're very fond of our nieces and nephews and do holidays with them and everything. But I'm just as married to my job as to Rick. I put in fourteen-, eighteen-hour days."

"What makes a good cop?"

"Empathy, if you can believe that."

"Explain."

"Not muscle. It's not like it used to be. I wish you *would* include this. We're not a frontier country anymore. Cops can't go around hitting people with nightsticks and assume that straightens them up. No more 'upside the head.' We need to be more professional. We need a wider variety of skills. The Special Weapons and Tactics, the Hostage/Barricade/Terrorist, the Heavy Weapons teams are such a small part of the job."

"They get the press, of course."

"They surely do. As a result, most cops lead lives of quiet desperation. Include this too: What we really need are people who can convince an elderly person to go to a cooling shelter when the temperature gets over a hundred degrees. People who can deal with abandoned children, win their trust. Specialists who can talk to angry teenagers and not make them worse. I used to *be* an angry teenager. I know this stuff. The old cops don't like this. They want to wade into a bar, whap a few people, and 'restore order.' The job is much bigger than that now and much more subtle."

"Like this whole horrible mess with Officer Jurack. My impression is he was very much an old-style cop."

She didn't respond.

I said, "Which makes it sad what's happened to Shelly Daniello and Chief McCoo."

"Mmm."

"McCoo has a good reputation among reporters."

"He has a good reputation with me, too."

"I don't think Daniello's case would have played out the same way with a male officer."

"I've never met Daniello."

"But you must know her record. Personnel is under your jurisdiction."

"I have twelve thousand current personnel records. I'm somewhat familiar with hers. I looked at it. But I don't know her personally." Still suspicious, she added, "Why are you so interested?"

"Interested? I'm *fascinated!* I'm not doing a story on it, I swear to you I'm not, but it's got elements that touch on everything that I personally care about. Her partner apparently didn't like being paired with a woman. Her brother-in-law was a bully. Her sister doesn't really support her, which reinforces all those complaints that officers have about domestic-violence calls—that the abused wife won't back them up. What's not to be fascinated with?"

She smiled. "Daniello, whatever she may have done at the Jurack house, was caught in a vise. She *had* to respond to the call. It's department policy. Once her brother-in-law saw it was her, she was in a mess. Abusive husbands often calm down in front of women cops. But in the case of a relative, I don't think so. He would be less likely to calm down, and far more likely to bluster, when he saw it was her. He'd think she was harmless. I don't know whether she fired when she didn't have to. I don't know whether she executed him. But I'd bet my shirt that he provoked it."

"Well, like I said, it won't go in my profile of you. Thanks. I think I have enough to use, Ms. Montoya."

"And you *will* let me see it?"

"Absolutely. Even when I'm doing something more investigative, I don't get my stories by lying to people."

"All right. I believe you."

"Does *Chicago Today* have an up-to-date picture of you?"

"I doubt it. Wait a minute. I've got one here." She pushed a button. Immediately, her secretary came into the room. "Henry, can you get one of my photos?"

"Yes, ma'am."

He was back in half a minute. She gestured at me and he handed me the photo. I looked at it, somewhat startled. The picture was unglamorous, a lot closer to the female version of Bob Cleary than the real woman was. I waited until he had left, and then said, "Ms. Montoya, I have to say this photo doesn't *begin* to do you justice."

A wry smile made her face look elfin. "Uh-huh. I had quite a time convincing the photographer to print the worst one, too. You'd have thought his artistic ethics were on the line."

"But why would you do this?"

"Most people don't know me. They see pictures. You think the city of Chicago is gonna let a good-looking woman control all those guns and squad cars and hardware?"

◆ 20 ◆

I am not superstitious. I do not believe in signs and portents. Nevertheless, when you've got luck running your way, why not jump on the bandwagon, or, as LJ might say, "There is a tide in the affairs of men, which, taken on the flood leads on to fortune."

So I walked right out of Deputy Superintendent Montoya's office and into Deputy Superintendent Bannister's anteroom. His secretary, this one a woman as pudgy and cheerful as Winter's was sour and birdlike, said, "Why, I'm sure Deputy Superintendent Bannister would *like* to talk with you. Let me see if he's free."

And he was.

Shakespeare is always right.

"Talked with Bob Cleary at the meeting this morning," he said, settling behind his desk. I was in a very nice leather chair, where he had courteously placed me before he sat down. Photographs on his desk of his wife and two pretty daughters at three different ages half-faced me. "He was being congratulated on the article you did about him."

"Well, I'm glad to hear that."

Paul Bannister was a wiry black man in late middle age. His hair was starting to show gray, but he was trim. Looking around his office, I saw running shoes peeping from under a long coat in his closet, so I knew how he kept the trim profile.

McCoo had told me Bannister had had a heart attack recently. Obviously, he was fighting back.

Bannister had asked his secretary to rustle up tea for us, giving me the option of green, black, or herbal. I wanted coffee, but naturally didn't say so.

I said, "I just finished interviewing Deputy Superintendent Montoya for tomorrow's paper. I want to use you the day after, if it's all right with you."

"No problem."

Bannister had been McCoo's mentor when McCoo was just coming on. Now he appeared to have turned on him, taking him off the Daniello case. There was no telling whether he had done it under pressure from the superintendent or whether he had suggested to Spurlark that it would be a good PR move. Bannister was the only African-American candidate for superintendent other than McCoo. Maybe McCoo was his closest rival.

I would keep my McCoo questions for later, until we had established a rapport. I said, "Tell me why you became a cop."

"Chicago was ahead of its time in getting African-American officers on the force. I was in high school, a Catholic high school in Chicago, trying to figure out what I was going to do next. And an 'Officer Friendly' came around talking about the department. Instantly, I thought, Wow! That's for me."

"Why?"

"Well, it was a respected position. And I think—when you're that age, you're pretty idealistic. You know how teenagers are."

"Not all of them."

"Most, I think. They have a nose for hypocrisy. That's why they're rebellious. They recognize two-faced behavior in their elders. They have an instinct, some of them, for self-sacrifice. Some become priests or nuns. At least they did in the old days. Or enlist in the army. Anyhow, I wanted to be a cop. You couldn't go on the force until you were twenty-one, but there was a kind of internship program—we were called cadets—and I took some community college courses while I was waiting, but the instant I turned twenty-one, I applied."

He told me a bit about his climb through the ranks. In telling it, he minimized what must have been real organizational ability, never mentioned the bias against African-Americans, never mentioned a past superintendent of ill repute who had said blacks couldn't handle leadership positions, and he said at least five or six times that he had been fortunate through out his career. He was very pleasant, and I just couldn't be sure how much ambition underlay the smooth and well-constructed exterior.

Finally, I asked, "Where does the department need to go now?"

"Technology. We need technology. We need a CAD system. Computer Assisted Dispatch. We need computers in all the cars for outstanding felony warrants. Think about this: Just having the fingerprint reader in all the district stations has streamlined things, saved us a *huge* amount of time, and made a lot of arrests possible."

"What is the fingerprint reader?"

"Say you're a patrol officer in a district. You arrest a person for shoplifting. You take him into the district station and the lockup person takes him to this box. It's got a monitor screen and a ground-glass plate. You roll his fingers on the plate as if you're making fingerprints, only there's no ink. The print comes up on the screen and the system tells you if you've made a good print or have to do it over. If all the prints are good, you beam it downtown and the AFIS—the Automated Fingerprint Identification System—here runs the print and, bingo, maybe you've got somebody who's wanted for a whole string of burglaries. This was never possible before. It was *extremely* cumbersome to send in prints. It was so time-consuming, you might have to let the suspect go before you even got results back. A real human being had to read them. That took man-hours, and time is money.

"We need computers in all the cars. We need instantly accessible data banks of child molesters. Rapists. All kinds of habituals. You get more service with existing personnel at a lower cost."

"What do you think makes a good police officer?"

"Professionalism."

The secretary brought in the tea. To real coffee drinkers, tea tastes as if you'd been raking leaves and you splashed some hot water on them.

Paul Bannister talked about how good it was for the department that women were on the force. "Having them there and having them work well has made it clearer to the public that policing isn't head-bashing anymore. Made it clearer to the department, too."

Aha! My opening.

I said, "There are people saying the Daniello case happened because she was a female officer."

"Oh, that's nonsense. Domestics are always dangerous."

"You don't think the fact that she was a woman made Jurack more defiant?"

"Not at all. I think men are likely to be more combative with men."

"Not just any men, though. Don't you think maybe wife abusers are more likely to ignore women officers?"

"That's a sociological question. I just don't know."

He was being cautious, and it didn't seem possible to push him to talk about Jurack. "I'm not writing anything on the Daniello case, sir. I just wonder whether maybe Jurack was one of those officers who should never have been a cop in the first place. I'm told he had a history of citizen complaints."

"I don't have that information."

Probably not true. He probably knew Jurack's whole work history, but not necessarily because of his direct department responsibilities. He'd know because top cops, like all cops, gossip. And he'd know from the emergency meetings they were having every day.

Bannister's divisions were Organized Crime, the Detective Division, Youth Services, and Auditing. He was McCoo's direct superior. Of all the top cops, he could have gotten the data from McCoo's office with the least fuss or suspicion. Still, he might have wanted it known that he *did not* have all of it, if there was a later search for the leak.

The whole thing was slippery; I couldn't put a firm hand on it anyplace.

I said, "Well, it's certainly worked out badly for Chief McCoo. He's had a very good reputation among reporters."

"Yes. And deservedly so."

Oh, come on, Bannister. Say a little more. Break your heart; grind out a whole sentence.

"The press says you took him off the Jurack case."

"It was a—uh—considered decision."

That was non-speak. I said, "This could end his career."

"I hope not."

A little time passed, but he didn't expand on the topic. I said, "Do you think we'll ever get to the bottom of what happened at the Jurack house?"

"I hope so. I have to say, Ms. Marsala, this is fairly far afield of your interview."

"Well, I can't help being interested. But you're absolutely right. It's not my subject. You saw the Cleary interview. I didn't print anything about Jurack in that, did I? Have I mentioned that if you want to see the interview before I send it in, I can fax it to you?"

He smiled then. "Cleary told us that you'd done that for him."

"So you can't really think that I'm going to extract information from you about Daniello and use it in the article."

"Well, I'll tell you, Ms. Marsala, there's a reporter in town who would. He'd write up the profile, and then a couple of days later he'd run the other parts of our discussion, and maybe skewed a little, too. And I don't doubt you know who he is."

"I can guess. And if you know who he is and I know who he is, and we both know his reputation, then you probably also know that I *don't* have that reputation."

He said nothing for a few seconds. He was at base an honest man, I thought, even though ambitious, and he did not enjoy being evasive. I sipped tea.

"My job is to make my areas in the department work," he said finally. "It's not to take on issues of staffing, or whether Jurack should have been a cop."

"But you are McCoo's direct superior officer. What happens in the Detective Division *is* your job."

He steepled his fingers.

"Part of making the department work is making it seem that it works. I don't mean that you just do cosmetic things. You have to get out the product, so to speak. The bedrock product. Patrol, arrests. Your investigations have to produce results. Your arrests have to be backed up by evidence that will stand up in court. McCoo's work is invariably solid. But beyond that the public has to have confidence in you; you also have to be *seen* to be doing these things."

"Which means . . ."

"If he can't prove to the public that he acted correctly, he's history."

See, you have to understand Chicago. Unfancy as the image is, sometimes I think of Chicago as being like a giant pizza. Chicago teems and bubbles. It is *not* slick. It is not polite. You can't get to know it without dripping and stringing and getting extremely involved with it. It is not nouvelle cuisine, all pretty, tidy, and in tiny little portions. Chicagoans have a degree of mutual respect for each other, which they demonstrate by giving each other a piece of their minds when they feel it's necessary to apply a healthful corrective. Chicago's a pizza with a slice for everybody. Chicago's got the hot pepper. It's got a few anchovies, and if you don't like them, you can

move a few blocks farther along. Chicago is a city of neighborhoods, and brags about it a lot. We've got the barbecue
here, and the pepperoni there, and the ground beef a little
farther on. Oregano. Salsa. Kimchi. Bean sprouts. Even
pineapple. We got the green pepper and the garlic, and
there's a corner for just plain. We've also got it all mixed
together in a lot of places, as if the delivery boy lost control
and it slid sideways.

What we have, I'm trying to say, is richness. Even if you
don't want to eat garlic every day, you kind of enjoy having it
available. It makes everything more interesting.

We have gypsies who came from Russia in 1900. Gypsies
from Serbia and Romania. Gypsies from Hungary who got
here in 1850 and moved into the northwest side.

Greeks on Halsted Street and now at Lawrence and West-
ern and still moving. Ukrainians. Lithuanians around Mar-
quette Park. First they worked for the Pullman Company
making train cars. Now they live in the suburbs.

Chicago Avenue way west was Sicilian. Taylor Street is the
old original Italian neighborhood.

Chinese came to Chicago in the 1800s and settled first
along Clark Street, from there moved on south to the present
Wentworth Street Chinatown area. Now there's a new Chinatown too.

Koreans far north on Clark.

And the CPD reflects all this diversity. Paul Bannister was
a real South Shore person. He had a kind of stately courtesy
and reserve that seemed to me characteristic of parts of the
area. The South Side has several middle- and upper-class
black neighborhoods. I knew Bannister to be from Chatham,
an area of large homes and wide, tree-lined streets. There are
deteriorated areas not far away, but you'd never know it in
Chatham.

Louise Montoya was a real Northwestsider from North
Milwaukee Avenue—tough, combative, extremely prag-
matic. Didn't expect to be handed anything on a platter. The

early Mexican migration to Chicago settled in South Chicago and Blue Island; then, like other ethnic groups, outgrew their neighborhoods and moved up Milwaukee Avenue.

Shelly Daniello was typical Chicago, too. Daniello said her father came from Taylor Street. He'd moved from there to the vast bungalow prairies of Chicago. He would have faced a certain amount of prejudice himself. Nobody remembers anymore, but two generations back, there was a quota at most colleges for Italians. Daniello herself might not even know that, but I'd bet her father would.

You don't have people apart from place. And place affects the people.

I love Chicago. You can really love a city. I don't mean just nostalgic love, just because you live there or used to live there and have fond memories. I mean love like you want to go out in the morning and walk just to see how the city has been doing since you saw it yesterday. Is it getting along all right? Its *moods* matter to you.

Because I love Chicago, I want Chicago to be okay. I find myself trying to fix things that aren't really my problem.

I phoned Shelly Daniello.

"Shelly? Can you meet me tonight at the Billy Goat Bar? In an hour?"

"Yeah. Why?"

"Why not?"

"I mean, has something come up?"

"No. I'm going to ply you with alcohol, get you liquored up, and find out what makes you tick."

· 21 ·

Among people who drink hard liquor at all, there are two main types, the Scotch drinkers and the bourbon drinkers. Scotch drinkers think bourbon tastes sickly sweet. Bourbon drinkers think Scotch tastes like distilled wood smoke and cringe at the thought of taking even a sip. I'm a bourbon drinker. Shelley Daniello was a Scotch drinker, but I wouldn't hold it against her. I'm as capable of being large-minded as the next bourbon drinker.

I'd written up my notes on the Montoya and Bannister interviews between four o'clock, when I left the CPD, and eight. I had typed at top speed, breaking only to munch peanut butter crackers and check the evening news. The Montoya piece was in rough but not embarrassing shape. The Bannister thing was truly rough. Channel Two's evening news had carried the story about McCoo's being removed from the Daniello case, and the news anchors had made it sound as if now, with him gone, maybe some progress would be made. Therefore I had left home highly crabby.

We sat far in the back of the Billy Goat. The tavern is below street level, and you can feel the trucks and El trains rumble overhead. Because the apartment I live in on Franklin Street faces directly onto the El tracks, I felt right at home.

"I'm paying," I said firmly to Daniello.

"Hey, you don't hear any complaint from me, did you?"

The waiter deposited our drinks and I told Daniello, "Drink up. Think of it as truth serum."

"I'm thinking of it as a fun evening out, if you don't mind."

She paused. "Not entirely, huh? In vino veritas, that sort of thing?"

"I have to break *something* loose. I'm floundering here."

"Not as much as I am. The round table is the day after tomorrow." Suddenly she looked sad. It wasn't an expression she often used, I thought, and her narrow, alert face wasn't especially suited to it. I felt stricken that I had to force her to relive the killing.

We both drank.

I very rarely drink much, not that I wouldn't like to. I don't relax easily, and I can see why people love liquor. But I work every night, reducing whatever notes I've made during the day to something I can understand later. You can't undertake two hours of serious chat with your word processor after a three-martini dinner.

When we had finished the first drink and ordered a second round, I got out my notepad and said, "This is what I want to do. I want to get a chronology of what happened, minute by minute, in that house."

"Okay."

Her willingness encouraged me. Maybe she wasn't guilty of executing Jurack. Maybe I could make everything be all right.

"Okay, start. You get the call on the radio." I didn't tell her I had heard the radio tapes and could check her version at several points.

"Uh—yeah. That was at fifteen thirty-one hours. Three thirty-one in the afternoon."

I wrote the time down. "Now you're driving to the 1764 Barcourt address."

"Right. You want times? We got to the address at three thirty-eight."

"Go back. You hear the call at three thirty-one. You're seven minutes driving over. When do you tell Hubner that it's your sister's address?"

"Oh, halfway there. Say three thirty-four, three thirty-five."

"Go on."

"We stopped two buildings down. This is standard. You want to slide up on 'em and see what the situation is before you go in. More so at night. This was bright day and kids running and yelling outside on their way home from school, but still you follow procedure."

"Okay. You walk to the main door of the apartment building. It's what time now?"

"Say three thirty-nine."

"You didn't have one of you go in the back and another in the front?"

"We heard screaming from all the way out on the street. Screaming sounds different when it's real. Marie didn't sound angry, she sounded agonized. So I scrambled."

"Okay."

"I had *told* Brad the layout of the apartment as we went to the door. That idiot! I run in and while I'm running in, I hear a bump. I know now that he'd run into the wall, but I didn't know it then. I surely didn't know he'd practically broken his nose and wouldn't be any good as backup. I thought he was right behind me."

"Give me a time."

"Well, from the time we parked until we ran in the door? Thirty seconds."

"Okay."

"Did I tell you before that I noticed the cat? The cat ran out when I opened the door. Ran out like the old saying, like a scalded cat."

"No, you didn't. Is that important?"

"We're taught that a lot of times if a husband goes on a rampage and plans to kill the whole family, he kills the dog or cat first."

"No kidding!"

"True. Anyway, the cat was fine. Actually, I guess I didn't tell you before. Funny. I don't think I've even thought about the cat until this minute. Maybe I underestimated Jurack at first because of that. Anyway—" She gulped half the drink in two swallows. "Anyway, I heard them in the back. I crossed the living room into the kitchen—"

"Quickly or slowly?"

"Pretty quickly. Cat or no cat, from the sounds I heard I was getting scared he was killing her. We're told to stop and listen. Then go a few feet farther and stop and listen again. We're told that we can't help the victim if we get killed ourselves. But when it's your sister, it's different. It can't have taken me even a whole fifteen seconds to get from the front door to the television room."

I wrote that down.

"Now I'll try to give you times for the rest of it." Her eyes took on a thousand-yard stare. She was watching the scene.

"Okay. I step into the television room. Marie's screaming. Immediately I see the light glinting off that blade, even before I realize Marie's been stabbed. Now when I see the knife, I know it's really serious. She's still screaming. I yell, 'Knife,' so that Hubner will know we've got an armed man."

"You never told me that before, either."

"Didn't I? Well, it didn't matter much. Hubner wasn't there. Anyhow, that took maybe ten seconds, tops, what I just told you. Now we got me and Jurack yelling at each other. 'Put down the knife!' Or 'Stop! Freeze!' All that. He says I won't have the nerve to shoot. At most a full minute. Then he lunges at me. I fire once. Cat, I am still totally convinced I fired when he was three or four feet away."

"All right. I understand."

"Shooting him took maybe three seconds," she said bitterly.

"Um-mm."

"Did I tell you I was pulling my gun while we were screaming at each other?"

"I don't remember."

"There's this training video we see that shows how far you have to be from a guy with a knife to get your gun out before he stabs you. You'd be surprised how far. If he's ten feet away, he can lunge at you and kill you before your gun has even cleared the holster. You have to have fifteen feet between him and you to get your gun out and more like twenty feet to get it clear enough to actually fire it."

"So you had it out."

"You bet. As soon as I saw the knife. Let's see. Where were we? I fire. He goes down kind of slowly. Maybe eight, ten seconds. Seems like a lot when it's happening."

"I can imagine." Now I took a large swallow of my drink. I could picture her watching with combined horror and relief as she realized Jurack was mortally wounded.

She said, "That must have been when Beanbag came into the room." I didn't respond to this. All the evidence, every single bit, was against her. "I heard a sound like a gasp or sob and looked over to my right and there she was against the wall, with one hand up to her mouth. I maybe took a half step toward her. But she came closer." Daniello put her hand over her mouth for a moment.

"This part is hard for you."

"I don't know what to say. I killed her father. I would *never* have shot him in front of her. I'd have let him kill me first, I think. Sometimes I wonder how she'll feel about me as she grows up. Will we ever get over this—as a family? Will she hate me?"

"I don't know. I wish I could reassure you."

"So. Call all that maybe fifteen seconds. No, maybe twenty. I was just so appalled that she was there. I stared at her. Then I turned back to the—um—body. Did I say Hubner came in around then, too, just as I was turning back to see whether Jurack was—uh, you know, alive or dead or what?"

"Yes."

"And there's my sister gulping and dithering and Hubner on the radio calling for an ambulance, and Beanbag saying, 'Daddy.' I mean, my God!" She stopped and drank again. "It was all over by three fifty. Do you need anything more? Isn't this enough?"

"Yeah, sure. It's enough." I closed the notepad. Daniello herself gestured for a third drink. I wasn't half done with my second. I shoved a bowl of peanuts closer to her, but she didn't take any.

I said, "So how are you and Marie getting along?"

"I keep telling her to get her act together. I'm impatient with her. I know I shouldn't be, but somehow gutless people just bother me. I mean, we had a call about a month ago. Woman heard a prowler. We go screamin' in—I mean, you don't want somebody to get killed while you're meandering slowly over to a call. So we go in and she's describing what she heard, and it just doesn't make sense. The prowler tapped on the window and peeked in at her, but I look out and the window's eight feet above the ground. That kind of thing. And after a while I ask her, maybe she thought she heard a prowler because she's alone there. Well, I didn't say it in so many words, and neither did she, but she almost did, what it really was—it was she was so lonely that she called the police. For company. For somebody to talk to! And in a way I've gotta sympathize, but in a way I don't. We talked to her for a while, but we've got other stuff to do. So I said to her there was this women's shelter in the neighborhood, women and their small children living with them, and the women going out working; they need people to go over and read to the children, maybe play games. You don't have to be qualified. Volunteers drop in, people from the churches in the area. So I tell her about this, figure she could meet people that way. 'Oh, I couldn't do that!' I mean, she's lonely, but she expects people to come to *her.* That bothers me."

"I see what you mean. And Marie?"

"That's like Marie. She's not gonna do anything to help herself. She's gonna get nearly killed. She put Beanbag in danger. But now I've done what I had to, and she's like, 'Oh, you should have stopped him but you shouldn't have killed him!' I mean, give me a break. Give me a goddamn break."

She drank half of her third Scotch and soda. I had let the waiter take my second drink away with an inch left in the bottom and nevertheless I was feeling warm and fuzzy. I sipped the new one cautiously.

"What happens next?"

"With my case? Sheer hell. They adjourned the round table to gather more evidence. Now they've got it. I mean, none of the autopsy stuff or the lab stuff was in for the first one. The expanded round table Monday will have Deputy Superintendent Bannister doing the questioning, I think, and somebody from the IAD, and my commander. And the FOP lawyer presumably defending me."

"What can they do to you?"

"Anything they want. They have a choice of three possible findings: 'exonerated,' 'unsustained,' or 'sustained.' Boiled down, they could keep me on the job and say I did right; keep me on but without a resolution, keep me but caution me; or they could fire me. At the very worst, they could recommend criminal prosecution."

"You say that very coolly."

"I'm not cool. I'm terrified. But there's just nothing I can do. Not one goddamn thing. I've thought about it and thought about it, but it happened the way I remember it. I truly believe you're trying to help. I think McCoo would help, too, if they don't destroy him first. But I know something else. They're gonna get me. They have all the power. This is a big media case and they need a scapegoat. They'll get me sooner or later, somehow or other, no matter what anybody does, and they're gonna destroy me."

"Maybe not."

"Maybe so. And you know, Cat, I'm just not the victim type. I don't know how to be a punching bag. I'm not any good at this." Her eyes glittered, but no tears spilled down her cheeks.

"It's absurd to blame you! He'd been beating your sister for years!"

"They'll say that's no reason to execute him. Spousal abuse is not a capital offense."

"But they can't possibly prove you intended to kill him—
that it was premeditated, I mean. That it was a murder. At
most you don't remember a few details."

"Hitting him with my gun and then executing him isn't just
a detail."

I decided to test her. "Suppose you said, 'Well, yeah. He
may have been closer than I thought. I waited to fire until the
very last minute.' "

She looked at me over her glass, her eyes serious. "You
mean, lie?"

"Couldn't your memory be wrong?"

"I don't think so. I remember it the way I remember it.
Even saying I don't *quite* remember would be lying, wouldn't
it? And I don't think I'm any good at lying."

"No. I don't suppose you are."

"Plus, even if I'm not criminally prosecuted, things aren't
gonna be the same. Not unless I'm proven innocent. One way
or another, if they want to get me, they can get me."

"Like how?"

"Suppose it's held 'not sustained.' A lot of the guys in my
district, my fellow cops, will still think I killed a cop for just
'chastising his wife.' Which they think is a perfectly normal
activity. Some of them think like that."

"Some guys everywhere think like that."

"Some of them really laid into me before I left. There were
a couple who kept calling me 'killer' and laughing. One of
them called me 'the avenger.' "

"But when you go back, what could they actually do about it?"

"Well, like, anonymous complaints to the IAD. 'I think I
saw Daniello take money from a drug dealer.' Whatever. Somebody makes a complaint, they're obligated to investigate it."

"Well, sure. That's as it should be. But at worst they'll find
it not sustained."

"Don't you realize how long that takes? Six months minimum. I've known cases that dragged around for two years.
And during that time you're frozen."

"Frozen?"

"No promotions, no nothing. Say you want to get into another unit. The tac team. I'd like the tac team. Or say I want to take the detectives exam. I've been thinking a lot about that. While you're under investigation, nothing happens. You don't get promoted. They could freeze me in place for *years* if they kept putting in complaints."

She paused. Then she added, "It won't come to that. The round table is gonna destroy me."

We spent another several minutes looking for consolation at the bottom of a glass. I had slowed way down, but she ordered a fourth. She was visibly loosening up, swinging her glass to emphasize what she was saying. Her eyes glittered with the mellowness of plenty of Scotch, unless it was her unshed tears.

She said, "The police department is the world's biggest boys' club."

"But Chicago has a lot of women officers."

"Yeah. And I don't doubt things are better than they were. But if you're a female, you're proving yourself constantly."

"Like showing you can be brave?"

"Showing you can fight. You know guys. You get in a real fight, defend yourself, beat some guy up, rip up your uniform, get bloody, dirt on your face, then you're one of the guys."

"You like that?"

"I understand it. You make a kind of unholy bargain when you join the cops. You're one of them. Or you're not. If you're really going to be one of the gang, you go along with what they do. You see somebody steal, you don't rat on him. You know there's brutality, you don't rat on the guys doing it. It's sort of a holy bargain, too, because they save your ass on the street and they get behind you when you screw up."

"What if the brutality gets really bad?"

"It's not easy to know what to do. If you speak out, they'll know. Even if it's anonymous. There's just too many ways to guess who was at the incident who would talk. Being on the

job, there's the people inside and the people outside. Outsiders don't know what goes on inside."

"It's kind of like marriage."

"Mmmm. Yeah, well, in a way that's right."

"Do cops have bad marriages because they're married to
the job?"

"They say so. But there are a lot of jobs like that. Surgeons.
Pediatricians. Politicians. Trial lawyers. I get impatient when
guys in my unit say naturally they've got wife trouble, they're
a cop. I mean, get a life. The spouse should get a life, too, for
that matter. People ought to be strong enough so you don't
have to hold their hand every minute."

"But you're not married."

"Well, yeah. It can be real hard to find somebody who
doesn't want his hand held."

At 11 P.M., we stood on the sidewalk. The temperature was in
the high fifties. March had come in like a lamb and was still
lamblike. Weird.

Daniello asked where my car was.

I said, "No car. I'm walking. I figured if I was going to be
drinking, the least I could do is not drive. Le'me get you a
cab. Or is your car around here?"

"Naw. Walked."

"You didn't drive?"

She said, "Hell, no. All I needed was to stack a DUI on top
of my other troubles. I figured if I was gonna be drinking, the
least I could do is not drive."

"You're my kind of person!"

"My buddy!"

"My pal!"

• 22 •

Daniello had drunk more than I had, but she held it better. By the time I bid her taxi good-bye and walked the last three blocks home, I was tacking a bit against a nonexistent wind. This was not how I liked to feel. It better have been worth it, but I wasn't sure it had been.

As my building hove into sight, three figures were visible sitting on the front steps. Tracy, Fred, and Russell.

"Whoa! Look at that. The three monkeys," I said. Russell was Hear-No-Evil, fingering his injured ear, although the bandage was now off. The ear was red and part of the upper rear portion was missing.

If Russell was Hear-No-Evil, Tracy was Speak-No-Evil, with her chin resting in her cupped hands. Fred had been leaning back with his eyes closed, See-No-Evil, if you stretched the concept.

Russell said, "We have to talk to you."

"How long were you gonna sit here if I didn't show up?"

"We got here at eleven fifteen," Tracy said. "We were giving you until twelve."

"Well, come on in."

The little party trooped up the stairs.

Mr. Ederle heard us, and when we reached the second floor, he popped open his door. Mr. Ederle is close to eighty, and frail. He never slept well, I knew, but his being dressed and up this late seemed extreme. I said, "What's the matter?"

"What's the matter? What's the matter! We're going to be thrown out on the street!"

"What?"

"Mr. Whillis was here today."

"I know that."

"He showed my apartment and yours, and I don't know who else's. And he said he liked it—"

"Who said?"

"The man Mr. Whillis brought around. He said he liked your apartment and mine both and he had a friend who might like to rent mine if he takes yours!"

"Oh, hell!"

"What are we going to do?"

"Let me think about it, Mr. Ederle."

"But I can't afford any more money."

"Neither can I, Mr. Ederle. It's sort of surprising to me that Whillis could get more than we're already paying for noisy apartments facing the El like this. Let me think about it. I'm, ah, just a little tired right now."

"Yeah, yeah, I know. I used to drink my dinner too, sometimes, if I was upset. Back when I could afford to. Which isn't anymore. Good night."

"The man's sharp as a tack," I said as I led my little party up the third flight of stairs to my floor. "He's living on a fixed income and his rent problem is real."

I unlocked my door—only two bolts, not excessive for the world today, and let my guests in ahead of me. Long John Silver, who had heard us coming as Mr. Ederle had, screeched angrily from his cage in the bedroom. He hates to be caged, and he also hates to have me get home late. By now he was one hot and spicy parrot.

"Excuse me a minute." I went into the bedroom and let him out. He squawked at me and flew into the living room, a distance of at least ten feet.

"Oh, wow!" Tracy cried.

Fred Koy said, "My grandmother has a parrot, but hers is—uh—mmm—"

"Prettier?"

African gray parrots are not pretty, no matter how much you like them. They are a gunmetal color with splotches of what looks like dried blood on the tail. The tail is stumpy and ungraceful. But they're the best talkers in the bird world. Usually. This time Long John said, "Braaaakkk!"

"Long John, please leave me alone. I've got guests."

He said, "Tell Ma dinner Saturday is fine."

"That's not what I said to Teddy. I said, 'I'll let you know if I can make dinner on Sunday.' "

"Tell Ma dinner Saturday is fine."

"You're much more accurate when it's Shakespeare talking. Although, come to think of it, I suppose the way I say something isn't as important as how Shakespeare says it."

"Tell Ma—"

"Oh, be quiet!"

He flew to a curtain rod and sat there, sulking. Fred said, "My grandmother has had her parrot forty years. How old is this one?"

"I think he's about forty-five. His name is Long John Silver. He was brought up the Mississippi by the captain of a shrimp trawler who thought it would be nice to retire to Chicago. Actually, the captain thought there was no water here and was quite surprised when he found out that Lake Michigan was so big you couldn't see across it. After he died, Long John was adopted by a professor of English from Northwestern University, who used to rent the apartment Mr. Ederle has now. Lived with him for twenty years, until he got into a scandal with a woman and had to move to Calgary—the professor, not the parrot. So I inherited Long John. The professor taught Shakespeare and apparently only spoke to the damn bird in the words of the Bard."

Tracy said, "So he's highly educated."

"And old," Russell said.

Conversation lagged for a few seconds. I said, "Anybody want something? Tea? Coffee? Personally, I am going to have a large glass of water with ice."

"Good for me, too," Russell said.

"I'll help," Tracy said, and she followed me out to the kitchen. We quickly filled four glasses with water and ice, not talking much.

When we got back to the living room, I said, "Now what—" but then an El train rushed by at express speed and there was no point talking until it was past.

"It's just lovely to have you here, guys," I said when quiet had returned, "but is there some special reason?"

Then Long John Silver imitated the El train.

"I thought he quoted Shakespeare," Russell said.

"Mostly Shakespeare. His repertoire is increasing. He does the El train and the phone ringing. And he's really good at the bathtub water gurgling down the drain."

Another silence.

"Listen, guys," I said. "Just exactly what is going on?"

Russell said, "Well . . ."

"We sort of . . ." Fred said.

". . . thought you might be able to . . ." Tracy said.

". . . help us out with a problem," Russell said.

"You're not the three monkeys, you're Hewey, Dewey, and Louie. Fred. You tell me."

"There's something wrong with McCoo."

"Wrong how?"

"I wanted to tell you yesterday when you were there, but we got interrupted. Do you remember he asked me for a formset? And I told him it was on his desk."

"Vaguely."

"Well, I'd already taken it in and told him here it was and he said okay."

"Everybody gets distracted now and then."

Tracy chimed in. "He does it more than now and then. He does it all the time, and it's not like him."

"That's true," I said. "He's usually on top of every detail."

Fred said, "I think it's just stress, but it's sure happening a lot."

"It's not just stress," Russell said. "I was afraid maybe the bomb had . . . um . . ."

"Russell's afraid the boss has brain damage," Tracy said firmly. But her eyes looked tight and worried.

"It's not brain damage," Fred said. "It's short-term memory loss."

"I think it's just stress," Tracy said.

"But it's definitely interfering with his work. We have to watch out for him all the time." Russell shook his head.

Tracy said, "We're afraid he'll make a mistake when we're not around to help."

Russell said, "Look, Cat, he's under a lot of pressure already. Suppose he drops the ball in public? Or when he's talking with one of the top cops? If he forgets some important point in a situation like that, they're apt to think he's hiding something."

Fred said, "Or lying."

I said, "Darn right. It doesn't matter whether he's stressed out or has some aftermath of the concussion; either way he could look evasive."

We sat sipping our ice water, like a meeting of the Women's Christian Temperance Union.

"Maybe we could call his wife and get her to keep him home a few days," Russell said.

"No, I don't think that would help," I said. "If he's not there, it'll look like he's staying away to avoid criticism."

"Maybe she could get his doctor to tell him to stay home."

"I don't think that'll work either. It's not the kind of job where you bring in a note saying you were really sick."

"Unless he's actually in the hospital," Tracy said. "Maybe I could talk his wife into getting their family doctor to admit him."

I said, "If you do, the department is gonna say he's too sick to do his job. And right now even that would be bad. I mean, they're on the verge of replacing him as it is. Just for show. Give them any excuse and out he goes—"

She said, "I see what you mean."

"Well, what *can* we do?" Fred asked.

We sipped some more ice water. We were a wild lot.

Should I tell them my suspicion that Bramble might have been the leak? And that McCoo and I had discussed it? No, not a good idea. First of all, I didn't want to sully Bramble's memory until I was sure. She might have had nothing to do with it. But second, it was possible that one of these people was the leak, not Bramble. Bramble had more contact with all the files, and yes, it would have been less noticeable for her to pull out and copy confidential data. Bramble was the only one besides McCoo who knew virtually everything that was going on. And yes, Bramble had been killed. But I didn't feel I had gotten even close to the bottom of what was happening and it was no time to give away my suspicions unnecessarily.

I said, "We just have to work harder, that's all. One of you is always near McCoo, right?"

"Well, yeah, until he goes to a top-cops meeting in the superintendent's office, and then he's on his own."

"But he doesn't routinely attend those meetings, right? Ordinarily it's just the deputy superintendents and the counsel and whoever. Right?"

"Yes, but they're worried about this case. They're meeting every two minutes, almost. They'll call him in again."

I said, "Have you warned him that he's having memory lapses?"

"Oh, Lord no! He might get mad," Tracy said.

"All right, then let's get moving. I need to know more about the people involved. Could Daniello's partner Hubner be lying? Who can get me Hubner's work history? Russell, you do most of the personnel work—"

"Right," Russell said. "I can have it for you tomorrow. Or Fred could. It's Fred's scheduled day, but we'll all probably go in and help."

"All right. If Hubner's lying that Belinda was in the room, I'd like to know why. Besides his work history, I'd like to know whether he's had serious trouble working with women officers."

"I'll see what I can find," Russell said. "Any serious complaints. But just gossip is going to be harder—"

"And what about Jurack? He had a history of excessive force complaints. Were any sustained?"

"I worked up that material for the boss already," Russell said. "It's not great. He'd had three sustained complaints."

"Why did they keep him?"

"You can't just fire a cop."

"But, Russell, if he had a history of abusing people—"

"Look, we have a union. We have rights. You can't simply fire a police officer. If a cop has four brutality complaints over five years, he's sent into the Behavioral Alert Program."

"Which does what?"

"Counseling. Retraining."

"And puts him back on the street?"

"Yup."

"What was Jurack doing to get these excessive force complaints?"

"Bringing in suspects that looked more banged up than necessary."

"And that's not serious?"

"Only three were sustained. Cat, people complain all the time. You can't go by just the complaints. You can have a lot of complaints, but they may evaporate when they're investigated. And if the complaint is not sustained, it doesn't go into your record against you. It's only if you get a certain number of *sustained* complaints that you can be fired."

"And I don't suppose they're easy to prove."

"Would you believe it if two drug dealers said some cop had been abusive to a third drug dealer? I mean, a lot of bad guys know how to use the system too. They scream 'abuse' to cast doubt on the cases against them."

"I suppose."

Tracy said, "The department tried to start a program a few years ago to identify problem officers. They had a software program, one that was developed for other things, like predicting the stock market."

"Brainmaker," Fred said.

"And they took a control group of officers who had been fired. Looked at a number of categories like AWOP days—absent without permission—years employed, education, insubordination incidents, traffic accidents, substance abuse, marital status, a lot of things. You assign their results a score of one point zero. Then they scored other officers who were still on the job on these categories, to try to predict who might turn into a problem."

"Did it work?"

"Who knows? The FOP had a fit. 'What's the cutoff number?—Zero point nine? Zero point ninety-nine?' 'Where's the research?' 'Where's the proof?' The department's using it but not talking much about it as far as I know."

Russell said, "Even a cop with a bunch of abuse allegations—don't you think he's entitled to a fair hearing?"

"Certainly. But he's not entitled to a job."

"But he is entitled to due process. You can't just take his job away."

"This isn't an ordinary job. I don't think an airline pilot is entitled to make a lot of mistakes. Not even a lot of little mistakes, because someday he may make a big one. A surgeon isn't entitled to his job. It's a privilege, not a right. And I think the same is true of police officers. You send somebody out there on the street with a gun and a license to shoot, and that's a privilege, not a right. He looks like he's making mistakes, he should be out of there. Don't you think so?"

"Oh, hell, yes. But you can see the other side."

Tracy said, "I'm not so sure I see the other side."

I said, "Guys? What exactly did you come here for?"

"We want you to tell McCoo," Russell said.

Tracy said, "You aren't an employee . . ."

"So we want you to tell him that he's screwing up . . ." Russell said.

"And tell him to be careful," Fred concluded.

They left by midnight, which was a good thing. I needed bed. I faxed the Montoya interview to the paper, and made some minor improvements in the Bannister piece. Montoya would run in the morning. I laid my woozy head on the pillow. As I turned out the lights, Long John said, "Tell Ma dinner Saturday is fine."

"Not now. This has been a very difficult day."

"When sorrows come, they come not in single spies but in battalions."

· 23 ·

A headache is nature's way of telling you that you need more caffeine.

I got up early on Sunday, despite feeling less than my usual high-octane morning personage. I become high-octane only on high-octane coffee. I tried to think of what good events this day could bring. I had a lunch/brunch scheduled with Sam, my new possible romantic interest. That ought to cheer me up. The interview with Montoya would be in the paper this morning. And I'd get paid for it, too.

But, in fact, I was depressed. Everything I had done up to now had not helped McCoo one whit. What good was I? All the work had been useless, and what was even more frustrating was that I would eventually have to give up spending so much time on McCoo and earn some more money. Every hour I spent on his problem put me farther in the hole. If I didn't make some money soon, I would be thrown out of my apartment, parrot and all, and would either have to sleep on the street with a Shakespeare-quoting bird or marry John. Or Sam.

Hmm.

I started the water for coffee before putting on the morning news. Long John Silver flew down from the curtain rod and sat on my shoulder.

"—a change early in the week. The unseasonably warm weather is expected to give way to rainy and cold, with a chance of a little snow—"

While the co-anchors joshed about the forecast of "white stuff," I poured water over the coffee.

"The mayoral race heats up as dark-horse candidate Chester Malling picks up the endorsement of Near North Side alderman Sonny Lippman," said Laura Chin, Channel Two's anchorperson. "Meanwhile Halliby is denying allegations that he—"

Malling, it seemed, had accused Halliby of accepting undocumented moneys for the campaign. "Undocumented" probably meant cash, probably untraceable cash. The big question now was who from. If Halliby dropped out, he and Malling would not split the vote, Malling would likely win, the mayor would lose, and then Superintendent Spurlark would be history for sure.

"And the ongoing investigation into the shooting of one police officer by another heats up as well. Chief of Detectives Harold McCoo has been removed from the case and the case given to a specially appointed task force—"

Damn! They already said that on the evening news. Why beat it into the ground?

"—and Assistant State's Attorney George Sheets has told Channel Two that he is considering seeking an indictment against Chicago police officer Shelly Daniello in the shooting death of her brother-in-law, Officer Benjamin Jurack."

Cut to a clip of ASA Sheets:

"We may have to let a jury decide this case," the state's attorney said, looking windblown but courageous in the plaza outside the Daley Center. The Picasso sculpture was behind his left shoulder, linking him with Chicago art and commerce through the ages. "There are too many different groups with different agendas dealing with this very sad case. If the department round table doesn't get to the bottom of what happened to Ben Jurack, it may be time to let the people decide."

"Damn!" I said, angrily killing the news with the remote. I pounded the sofa with my other hand. "Damn! Double damn!"

"Wraaawk!!" Long John said, flying up into the air, shedding feathers.

"Oh, I'm sorry, baby, I'm sorry! It's not your fault."

But he just sat on the curtain rod, looking reproachfully at me out of the eye on the right side of his head. Then he swiveled his head a hundred and eighty degrees and looked out of his left eye. Apparently the two views of me were equally bad, because he said "Wraaawk!" again.

Gray feathers slowly surfed the air down to the floor at my feet.

"I'll make it up to you. I have a banana."

This is LJ's favorite food. Banana must be a sort of parrot chocolate. He followed me into the kitchen. While I peeled the top third of the banana to give him, he said, "Tell Ma dinner Saturday is fine."

I stood stock-still for a couple of seconds. Then I blinked and smiled.

"Oho!" I said. "Why, that little devil. Thank you, LJ, for the idea."

He cocked his head.

"You've earned the entire banana. Go for it. Knock yourself out."

When I saw Mr. Whillis on the second-floor landing, in conversation with Mr. Ederle, I was delighted. Maybe this was going to be a really good day after all. Mr. Ederle was close to tears. Not for long.

"Good morning, sir," I said to Whillis.

"Have you made a decision yet, Ms. Marsala?"

"Yes, I'm staying. So is Mr. Ederle."

"Fine. I will expect the increase to start with the May first check."

"No, no, Mr. Whillis. Mr. Ederle and I plan to stay here at our present rent. And you should be happy, since you don't have anybody else who wants the space."

"I have my client from yesterday. Mr. Ederle here met him. And he has a friend who's interested."

"Your client is a shill, Mr. Whillis. He's either your brother or your brother-in-law."

His mouth fell open, but being a greedy man not used to giving anything away, he instantly closed it. "That is not true."

"Oh, yes, it is. When you were in my apartment, he told you that your mother was expecting you for dinner Saturday."

He gaped at me as if I were psychic. Weakly, he said, "No, he didn't."

"Yes, and since you don't have any real prospects for the apartments, I don't even mind telling you how I know. My parrot quoted him as saying, 'Tell Ma dinner Saturday is fine.' Now, that had me confused for a while, because I had told my own brother that we could go to our mother's on Sunday."

"Well, that's what your bird heard, then."

"No, we call her 'Mom,' not 'Ma,' and we weren't going on Saturday."

"So the bird made a mistake," Whillis said.

"Oh, no, you don't! This is a parrot who can remember Henry the Fifth's entire rousing Crispin Crispian speech to his troops before the battle of Agincourt, when he hasn't heard it for at least ten years! A little thing like Saturday or Sunday is not going to confuse him."

"You can't prove that."

"I don't need to prove it. I can call your bluff. Your rent check will be in the mail. For the usual amount."

Mr. Ederle smiled.

Meanwhile, there was the catastrophe that was about to happen to Shelly Daniello.

I did not think that Daniello deserved to be indicted. But honesty told me she certainly did deserve a hard second look.

I had put aside some uneasiness about Daniello while drinking with her last night, but now the doubts came back to me. She had remembered the cat. The cat that wasn't dead, a variation on the dog that didn't bark in the night. This was supposed to have suggested to her that Jurack wasn't dangerous enough for her to be really cautious. It meant that it was okay for her to go rushing in ahead of her partner. But maybe she actually hurried ahead so that she could kill him unobserved.

Then there was her claim to have called out "Knife!" to Hubner. He had said he heard her call out, but hadn't told me that she said "Knife" specifically, as far as I could remember. I would have to look back at my notes on his statement.

Were these two recovered memories a little too convenient? Was she trying to put herself in a better light?

Sheets had said he was "considering" indicting Daniello. I had to see McCoo, and find out how much time we had in view of this new development. Did Sheets mean he would decide immediately after the round table tomorrow ended? Or that he'd wait a few days to see whether the idea flew well with the public? Whether the scandal petered out? Maybe he just hoped that the threat of an actual criminal prosecution would scare some of the participants into telling the truth.

I got into one of the antique CPD elevators. Five extremely large police officers got on with me. Two were administrators in semi-plainclothes—crisp blue shirts, sharply creased navy pants, shiny shoes, and gun. Three were walking hardware stores—guns, radios, flashlights, handcuffs, key chains, name badges, plus other tools of the trade on their belts. They'd have to strip to get through a metal detector. Since they all seemed to be seven feet tall, even though common sense told me they were probably only six-two, their equipment all stuck in my face or neck. If you are just over five feet, much of your life you feel like a fourth grader who's accidentally wandered onto the high school playground. Because it was Sunday, there were fewer of them around, so I wasn't crushed.

I wasn't supposed to be visiting McCoo. I got off on the fifth floor, where the top cops' offices were, all in a row. I was going to walk up the stairs to eight, McCoo's floor.

The superintendent's outer office was open. Well, no wonder. They had a crisis to deal with. I walked in for the third time, asked the secretary for an interview, was rebuffed for the third time, and left. Took all of a minute. As his secretary said, "They've got a meeting scheduled in an hour, Ms. Marsala. This is a very bad time."

The interview with Montoya had indeed been in this morning's *Chicago Today*. I hoped she was pleased with it. Maybe it was time to try again to talk with Gregory Dennison Winter, the Mercedes of the top cops. But I didn't feel like being rejected again. I just glanced in the door of his office as I went by. There was the bird lady, guarding the sanctum, even though it was Sunday—evidence of a real CPD crisis. Beyond her, in the inner office, Winter was again reading a newspaper. He saw me over the top of it.

Suddenly he stood. He raised his hand in an imperious gesture, beckoning me in. Puzzled, I went as far as the outer office, near the bird lady.

He came out to me and halfway there he amended the imperious gesture. The beckoning finger was abruptly joined by other fingers in a friendly flat-hand wave. His voice was pleasant as he said, "Aren't you Catherine Marsala?"

"Yes, I am."

"Well, I have to wonder, why haven't you come to me?"

"For what?"

"For an interview. You seem to have chosen to do everybody else."

I stared. How often had I come here? Three times? How often had I been turned down? Every time. And he'd seen me every time and heard me ask. I was about to say so, and to point out that bird lady had been curt every time, when I caught her eye. She didn't plead. She just looked at me, but I had to stop and think. What would it be like to work for this asshole?

"Actually, Deputy Superintendent Winter, I was planning to stop in this morning."

*   *   *

Tall, slender, wearing a three-piece suit, he showed me which chair I was supposed to sit in. He was straight-backed and had uncompromising, aristocratic features, if by aristocratic one means a long, bony head, thin nose, and high forehead. It was easy to imagine him as one of the judges in a witchcraft tribunal.

He did not object to my tape recorder, which I placed on the desk.

"You've read the profiles in *Chicago Today?*" I asked him.

A slight frown creased his smooth forehead. "I read this morning's." He didn't want to appear too much the pawn of publicity or the slave of the papers.

"I see."

He looked at me and I looked blankly back. I thought it would be interesting to see how he would begin. In McCoo's words, find out what was important to him, what he was selling. And anyway, dammit, he'd called me into his office. Let him make an effort.

All right, I was feeling crabby, irritable, pigheaded, and self-righteous. And it worked.

"My family never intended for me to be a peace officer," he said.

Personally, I think the change from "police officer" to "peace officer" is pretentious spin-doctoring, but I didn't say so.

I turned on my tape recorder.

"They wanted me to go to law school, and then enter the family business. My great-grandfather had established woolen mills and my grandfather expanded to include a chain of retail haberdasheries."

Oh, hell, are we going to hear the whole family history?

"They believed that legal training was the best foundation for business. It made a man think clearly. And, of course, with legal training I could better evaluate the tax laws, liability laws, and query any advice that our corporate lawyers might give us."

I took notes carefully, despite the tape recorder, as he worked his way from 1850 to 1965. At that point he graduated from law school.

"I was tired of business and tired of hearing about business. So I applied to the police department. My father was scandalized."

Now he's a rebel. "So what does he think now?" I asked.

"What?"

I'd broken his train of thought. "What does your father think now about your being a *police* officer?"

"Oh. Well. He's proud of me now, of course. But it took several years."

"I see. Why did you do it?"

"My feeling was that, if you have been financially blessed, you owe something back. This country has been good to my family. It was time one of us served our country in return. Not that the Winters haven't served in wars, of course, but . . ." He hesitated, not quite having figured out where this was going.

"You can't expect wars every day?"

Smile. "Well, that isn't exactly what I meant. I mean that there are ongoing social problems that we have to cope with."

"Why not run for office? The Senate, maybe?"

"Well, I could have, I suppose. It's very uncertain, though. You can't really manage public taste."

"No."

"A police department has a never-ending struggle with crime and a never-ending mandate to keep the peace and make the day-to-day lives of our citizens safe."

He stared pointedly at me until I wrote it down. Maybe, like me, he figured the tape recorder might fail and if so, his valuable words be lost.

"What ongoing social problems did you have in mind?"

"Crime, of course. Lack of moral values. The way things are today, we need police on the streets. I don't mean in squad cars, but on foot. Chicago has twelve thousand police officers. We need eighteen thousand."

"What would they do?"

"Hands-on proactive attention to the community. We need to go back to the days when the cop on the beat would give immediate chastisement."

"What—"

"In the old days, if the cop saw a bum steal an apple, he'd clip the thief with his baton. That's immediate. What we do now is arrest a guy, and we only do that if the offense is a big one, because the courts are swamped and the prisons are overcrowded. It takes months for him to go through the system, and in the end he's let off if the crime isn't violent, because there's only room for violent offenders."

"So you're saying the police should have the right to hit people?"

"Oh, they have the right already. In certain cases. Resisting arrest, for instance. Or if they see somebody attacking another person. I'm not talking about that. I'm talking about street punishment for smaller offenses. The populace needs directing."

He was being surprisingly frank. I've noticed this phenomenon all my writing life. It's not only that people relax with you after a while—though they do—and start confiding. The big element is simply that people mostly do what they think is right. They may be way off base about what's right. They may actually be foolish or cruel, but they think they're right. So they want to explain it to you. Convince you, if they think you disagree. Make a pal of you if they think you agree.

I once had a person tell me why he had to smother his father. I'm not kidding.

Winter would soon decide that he didn't really want this last remark in print. And personally, I didn't care. I was trying to guess whether he was a man who would leak confidential facts to the press or blow up McCoo's office.

Winter's smooth voice went on. I made squiggles while I

studied the plaques on his walls. Handball competitions. All-county champion. Awards for marksmanship. And—good heavens!—polo trophies from twenty years back. Polo. You don't get a lot of that in the city of Chicago. Photographs of two teenage children, a boy and a girl. No wife. I had heard Winter was divorced—nastily divorced.

"The people of Chicago really want the police to keep control. It's just difficult to come right out and say it. But you know, Miss Marsala, we have the same Constitution today as we had in the days when the police were *expected* to administer a little dollop of street justice."

"I'm as ambivalent about the police as anybody else," I said. "I understand what you mean. I want the police to pick up people who might mug me as I go about my work. I'm on the streets on foot a lot and out at night a lot, and I know what it is to be very, very uneasy."

"Well, you see."

"But when it comes to me, I expect them to have every part of the Bill of Rights firmly in mind."

"We all want *everybody else* to be policed."

"Right. We're quite sure we don't need it ourselves."

"Oh, well," he said, glancing at his wristwatch, which looked flat and gold and expensive, "we won't solve all the problems of the world today." He caught my eye again. "I'd just as soon you left out the part about street justice."

"I'm doing a profile. I don't need it."

"Good. Well, regretfully, I have a meeting in ten minutes. You will fax me the draft, like you did with Cleary and Montoya." Unaware that he had just told me he'd seen both profiles and talked with their subjects about me, he handed me his card. It included a home fax number.

"Cat, I have to tell you, you're going about this all wrong."

"Oh, thanks! All I needed was somebody else to tell me that."

"Wait a minute. I'm trying to help you."

"Everybody is trying to help me."

Sam and I were having Sunday lunch/brunch in a grape-purple booth in Tinseltown, a Hollywood-style restaurant with cinema icons all over. We must have been in the Lauren Bacall booth. Her picture hung above us and there was a button for service on the table that said "Just whistle." I pushed it. It whistled. Probably they'd have preferred to install an actual whistle, but the health department wouldn't have let them.

The interview with Winter had set me back an hour, which meant I had to rush over to my brunch with Sam. No chance to see McCoo. Just being exposed to Winter for sixty minutes made me hungry for something solid. One thing you have to say for food—it's honest.

When the waiter arrived, dressed like a film director in jodhpurs, Sam ordered the DeVito, stir-fried shrimp, and I ordered the Stallone, beef on two buns.

"Believe it or not, the food's good here," Sam said.

"I believe you. You're usually right."

I met Sam just a few months ago. I am coming to like him more than I like John, but I see him less, because of his schedule and mine. He's a trauma surgeon and works the evening shift at University Hospital. He has long hours, and also does some writing and teaching. When he has time off, I seem to be working. When I get a break, he's working. At least it's mutual.

"Listen, I'm right about this too," he said. "There really isn't any way you can tell which of the top cops is stabbing McCoo in the back."

"Somebody already told me that. I suppose you want me to just walk away from my friend."

"Absolutely not! That would be totally immoral. Plus, I don't think you could live with yourself."

"Oh."

"But I *do* want you to get a little more cold-blooded about this quest you're on."

"Oh?" I said suspiciously. "Exactly how?"

"Look. Think about my job, what I do. When a case comes into the trauma unit, there's usually more than one thing wrong with the patient and I have to make a fast decision about what to treat first. Prioritizing is probably the second most important thing I do, after diagnosing and before treating."

"Yeah. So?"

"So I certainly don't listen to the patient's opinion of the priorities. What you're doing is listening to McCoo."

"Naturally. He's my friend."

"I had a patient Friday afternoon who was injured in a construction explosion. Some dynamite went off too soon."

"That sounds horrible."

"Was. Anyway, my patient was rapidly going into shock. The concussion had lacerated his liver and he was bleeding in there someplace. The blast had also burned his face—first- and second-degree burns, superficial enough so they hadn't destroyed the nerves; he could feel them, and therefore he knew about it. So he was all worked up that he was going to look like the Phantom of the Opera. I mean, here's a guy who's going to die in thirty minutes if I don't do something fast and he's worried about cosmetics."

"So?"

"So I told him, sure we'll take care of the burns. Right away. But me, I didn't give them another thought. We went in, I tied off the bleeders and sent him to recovery, and about the time he wakes up somebody else will deal with his face. And the point is, I had to prioritize for him."

"All right. I understand."

"McCoo can't deal with life right now. He's not entirely rational. He's had too many blows. He's been accused of lying. His lifetime competence has been questioned. His close friend and aide has been killed. Another unidentified friend has betrayed him. He's been taken off the case because the superintendent doesn't trust him anymore. And he's had a very significant head injury. Of *course* he's not able to cope. You have to cope for him."

"He wouldn't like to think he was weak."

"He's *not* weak. What kind of person would he be, if all these things happened to him and he just shrugged it off? He'd be a psychopath, that's what. He's having trouble precisely because he's a good man. Don't forget that."

"I agree."

"See, he's most upset because somebody he knows and likes is trying to destroy him. That's very upsetting, of course. So that's what he asks you to investigate. But there's really no way that you can tell who it is by just talking to these top cops. You might guess, but even if you guess right, you wouldn't have any proof. Find the top cop is what McCoo wants, but it isn't what he needs."

"What does he need? To know whether the leak was in his office?"

"In a minor way. If the leak was Tracy, Russell, or Fred, McCoo should know because the leaks could go on."

"Right."

"But far more important than that, he needs to know what really happened at Jurack's house. If you could prove him right about Daniello, that would be the best thing that could happen to him. Even if McCoo is wrong, if you could prove

what really happened to Jurack, and that there was a reasonable explanation of why McCoo misinterpreted it, that would
be okay, too. What is killing him *politically* is the suspicion
that he not only was wrong but covered up for Daniello."

"That's true."

"You have to find what's killing him, like I do, and stop the
dying process, like I do. Let somebody else hold his hand
later about a friend betraying him. Don't do what he says. You
do what he *needs*."

"And what do I tell him?"

"I'm afraid, Cat, that for the time being you should tell him
whatever he wants to hear."

Tracy, Russell, Fred, and McCoo himself were all working at
file drawers when I walked in. McCoo was that kind of boss.
He didn't think he was too big and important to lend a hand.
It was one of the reasons they were all so loyal.

McCoo said, "The ATF has come up with something. They
say the letter bomb was hand-delivered."

"Really by hand, or department mail?"

"Not department. It had a postmark that looked good at a
casual glance, but was faked."

"Oh." I was disappointed. "That makes it harder to trace."

"Maybe. The FBI's working on the ink."

"Hmmm."

"Still getting straightened up?" I asked, looking around. "I
don't usually find you all here on Sunday."

"I didn't make 'em come in," McCoo said, smiling. He was
glad they cared.

"You knew they would."

"I'll let 'em go early."

"I'll believe that when I see it."

"They've been here since nine A.M." He turned to the
three. "It's one o'clock. Maybe you should get on home."

"Half an hour we'll be finished," Tracy said.

"How's it going?"

"Finally got all the pieces reassembled," Russell said.

"We've pretty much put stuff back together," Fred said. He stopped, swallowed, glanced at the place where Bramble's desk had stood, and couldn't help adding, "Except . . ."

Tracy said, "Don't!"

There was a pause, during which nobody spoke and they didn't meet each other's eyes. I let my gaze pass over them all, though. Fred Koy, Russell Lupinski, Tracy Shoemaker. Over the last twenty-four hours, because of the faked blood-alcohol sheet on Daniello, I had come to believe one of them was the leak. Not Bramble.

It wasn't only the alcohol report that made me think this. If Bramble was the leak, then our theory must be that the top cop had blown her up to silence her. There had to be easier ways of doing that. Pay her more. Threaten her. The top cop only had to keep her mellow for another few days, until the election. Plus, she wouldn't get her big reward until he became superintendent, whoever he was. This was no time for her to turn on him. If she was the leak.

But if she wasn't, it all made sense. She had an idea who the leak was, and she was getting ready to expose him. Or her.

Tracy, Russell, or Fred.

I hoped I wasn't letting my suspicion show in my face or voice.

After an awkward few seconds, I said, "McCoo, I shouldn't stand here in the main office. Somebody might walk in and see me. Let's go to your office. I've got time right now to go over that stuff."

"Superintendent Spurlark still won't give me an interview," I said to McCoo, while he opened his safe.

"Smart of him."

"He can see from what I've written that I'm being kind to these people."

"Cat, he knows he puts his foot in his mouth. He'd be better off if he gave up talking entirely."

McCoo had to check three pockets before he found the safe key in his inside breast pocket. On the one hand, that told me that he was still having memory lapses. On the other hand, it also told me that his cop instincts were in place. He'd kept the key in a safe place, even if he couldn't remember where.

"I'm looking for Bramble's March work schedule," I said, glancing at his open office door. We were talking softly, but I was uneasy. I held up my hand, then put my finger on my lips. I gestured at the door, and mimed closing it. He cast his eyes at the ceiling, so I just went over and closed the damn thing.

He said, "Did you have to do that?"

"I don't know, McCoo. I wish I did." I said, "Okay, now I'm looking for Bramble's schedule of who worked when."

"For this office?"

I snapped, "What other office would she schedule?" When he gazed sadly at me, I said, "I'm sorry. But I'm tense. Are you thinking, like I'm thinking, if Bramble wasn't the leak, it was Fred or Tracy or Russell?"

"God, I don't know. I just don't know anything anymore."

I remembered what Sam had said, and let the remark lie. I said, "I also need to separate out any newspapers or clippings on the Jurack case."

He nodded and we started to work.

"I'll do the staff calendar," I said. "You see if you can figure out when each piece of data that was ultimately leaked first arrived in this office. Jurack's head bruise, Belinda being in the room, and the distance between Jurack and Daniello."

We had dried most of the damp pages before we put them back in the safe, but still some had managed to stick themselves together. Also, Bramble had kept her office work schedule on a one-week-per-page loose-leaf calendar, so we had to find three different pages for the first three weeks of March. Then I discovered that the water damage had caused parts of the pages to stick to pages next to them. When I pulled them apart, either the calendar pulled off parts of the other pages, leaving extra globs of letters on the calendar, or the other pages pulled off patches of the calendar, leaving white areas.

It took me about an hour to reconstruct on a separate sheet of paper the schedule of work in McCoo's office. McCoo, meanwhile, was rummaging in his records.

I added who was actually in the office today and yesterday to Bramble's sheets, written many days ago. My final updated reconstruction of Bramble's calendar:

Staffing:

Saturday	March 8	Russell Lupinski
Sunday	March 9	Tracy Shoemaker
Monday	March 10	Shoemaker, Fred Koy
Tuesday	March 11	Lupinski, Koy, Shoemaker
Wednesday	March 12	Lupinski, Shoemaker
Thursday	March 13	Lupinski, Shoemaker, Koy
Friday	March 14	Lupinski, Koy
Saturday	March 15	Koy
Sunday	March 16	Shoemaker
Monday	March 17	Lupinski, Shoemaker
Tuesday	March 18	Lupinski, Shoemaker, Koy
Wednesday	March 19	Lupinski, Shoemaker, Koy
Thursday	March 20	Shoemaker, Koy
Friday	March 21	Lupinski, Shoemaker, Koy
Saturday	March 22	Lupinski, Shoemaker, Koy
Sunday	March 23	Lupinski, Shoemaker, Koy

Shelly Daniello had shot Ben Jurack on Friday, March 7, just before the beginning of this calendar. Today was Sunday the twenty-third. The bomb had exploded on the nineteenth, and that was why Russell Lupinski was not in the office on the twentieth. He was having surgery. Bramble had originally scheduled him to be at work.

Finally McCoo handed me his dates for the arrival in his office of the data: the autopsy protocol which told about the

head bruise, Hubner's statement about Belinda being in the
room, which arrived here in a day, since it had come out at the
round table, and the CPD lab info on the powder stippling. I
entered them onto a new, larger graph:

	Staff:		When info was received in McCoo's office:
Saturday	March 8	Lupinski	Hubner's report
Sunday	March 9	Shoemaker	
Monday	March 10	Shoemaker, Koy	
Tuesday	March 11	Lupinski, Koy, Shoemaker	autopsy report
Wednesday	March 12	Lupinski, Shoemaker	
Thursday	March 13	Lupinski, Shoemaker, Koy	
Friday	March 14	Lupinski, Koy	CPD lab results
Saturday	March 15	Koy	
Sunday	March 16	Shoemaker	
Monday	March 17	Lupinski, Shoemaker	
Tuesday	March 18	Lupinski, Shoemaker, Koy	
Wednesday	March 19	Lupinski, Shoemaker, Koy	
Thursday	March 20	Shoemaker, Koy	
Friday	March 21	Lupinski, Shoemaker, Koy	
Saturday	March 22	Lupinski, Shoemaker, Koy	
Sunday	March 23	Lupinski, Shoemaker, Koy	

I studied this and studied it until my brain fogged, but
nothing seemed to jump out at me. Finally, I said, "McCoo,
I'm going to the ladies' room. Do I need a key?"

"No. We have to have public bathrooms here because of
the courts here."

The outer office was deserted, which I supposed was a
good thing. I was tired of guarding my face around the staff.
For just a passing moment, I examined their desks. Fred's was
tidy, everything cleaned off the top except a closed-up laptop
and pictures of two children of Asian ancestry, both girls, I
thought, but so young that I wasn't sure.

Tracy's desk was also clean, but there were supplies on top. A jar of pencils and pens. A monitor and keyboard. A package of discs.

Russell's was a total mess. There was a leaning pile of manuals for various computer programs, as well as booklets explaining the use and care of a fax, a printer, a laptop, and several other types of equipment. Pens and pencils were scattered everywhere. Blank formsets had been left in piles. There was a stack of blank paper, some of it pink, some yellow, some white. Half of a granola bar lay near one corner.

Shrugging, I went out in the hall.

The bathrooms in the CPD building are functional at best. This one was very clean, because the courts on this floor are only in session Monday through Friday and the janitorial staff had been able to catch up with their mopping. Their mops and pails were stored in an alcove. Beyond clean, the only thing you could say for it was that it was dreary. It was gloomy, an interior room with no windows. Institutional fluorescent fixtures ran along the very high ceiling, but of four of them, one was out and one was flickering. A line of sinks with exposed pipes ran along one wall, a line of toilet stalls along the other. I went into a stall and closed the door.

Half a minute later, I heard the hall door open. Somebody turned on a water tap.

A minute later, I was finished with what I went there for and realized I heard the water still running. Well, maybe this woman, whoever she is, likes really cold water. Just before I left the stall I noticed something even odder.

I was having a hard time catching my breath.

Asthma? I didn't have asthma. Maybe there was a pollutant in the air. But as I opened the stall door I realized I was breathing perfectly normally. I felt no asthma-like struggle to suck in air.

It was the air itself that was wrong.

I burst out of the stall and saw, lying next to the sink, a halon fire extinguisher turned on. The running water had covered the hissing. Halon is for electrical fires, computer fires. It's a non-oxygen gas that replaces all the oxygen in a room. No oxygen, no fire.

I ran to the hall door and pushed hard, but it wouldn't open. Maybe it opened in. Yes, it did; the hinges were on the inside. I pulled. It still wouldn't move.

I turned, looking for a window to break, but there was no window. I couldn't breathe. A clock in my head said I'd been without oxygen for fifteen seconds. Sixteen. Seventeen.

I grabbed the halon extinguisher and tried to turn it off, but the turn-off slide had been removed.

Twenty seconds. Twenty-one. Twenty-two.

I pulled the door handle with my full weight. Again. And again. Panic and muscle force were using up what little oxygen I had left and the door only jiggled. It wouldn't open.

Thirty-one. Thirty-two. There were bright flashes of light in my eyes.

Forty seconds. I was starting to feel woozy. Should have built up my body aerobically. Should have jogged. Should have swum. Underwater. Lap swims. Forty-six seconds. There were dark dots in my field of vision. I pounded on the door. Somebody please come. Forty-nine. Fifty.

I dropped to my knees. Conserve oxygen. Stop panicking. Panicking uses oxygen. Hibernate. Wouldn't that be nice? Sleep awhile.

I fell to the floor near the door. Fifty-six seconds. Floor near the door. Crack under the door.

I put my mouth to the crack under the door, head on the floor, ear to the floor, and sealed the opening top and bottom with my lips so as to take in as little air from this room as possible. I blocked the gaps off at chin and forehead as well as I could with my fingers, and sucked in air.

Twenty minutes later, McCoo found me.

The door had one of those staple-shaped handles on the

outside. Somebody had simply stuck a broom through the handle and across the doorjamb. McCoo had pulled the broom out and opened the door tentatively—after all, it was the women's bathroom—saw me on the floor looking up at him, and said, "What happened?"

But he could see what had happened. McCoo took the steps a detective takes. He bagged the broom. He bagged the empty halon fire extinguisher. He called the First District and asked them to send up an evidence tech to fingerprint the door handle.

"You'll either find nobody's fingerprints or everybody's," I said.

He helped me back to the office and sat me down to rest in his desk chair. McCoo paced around the office making grunts of fury. Suddenly he pointed into the main office. "There! Look, it was our fire extinguisher!"

Sure enough, the bracket near the back of the main office was empty. It was the one he had not used the day of the explosion.

"You'll find everybody's fingerprints, then," I said.

"Goddammit!"

"I don't feel very well."

"You don't look so good, either. Let me take you to a doctor."

"Oh, no, no. I'm just queasy."

"I'm not going to let you go home this way. For all I know, that stuff may do lung damage."

"I don't have time to go to a doctor. I've got the Winter profile to write and fax off tonight."

"So I'll force you."

"Tell you what. Compromise. I'll call Sam as soon as I get home and ask him how dangerous the stuff is."

"Promise?"

"Yes, dammit! I promise."

"I'll call later to check."

"All right. All right."

"Good."

"You remember that chart we were working on? I know what it needs now, McCoo."

"What?"

"The time that each leak first appeared in the newspapers."

"It'll take a long time to work that out. The leaks got repeated over and over in all the papers. It means going through dozens of stories in dozens of papers, looking for the leaks, and then listing the dates."

He looked so weary, I said, "Well, you don't have to do it tonight. You go home, too. Get some rest."

"Maybe you're right. I'll do it tomorrow."

"Do it all by yourself. Don't let anybody in the office help you. Don't even tell them about it."

"No." He looked so beaten and sad, my heart ached. He got up, saying, "Let's go."

"Okay."

"And Cat, I'll walk you down, but I can't follow you around. You're obviously in danger. Watch yourself."

"Sure."

"I mean it. Sometimes you're such a macho—"

"Not this time."

The truth was, I felt sick and weak. Being smothered by halon isn't good for people. We locked the office safe. We locked his inner office. He took the keys with him as we walked out. I noticed he glanced at the desks, as I had earlier. He said, "One of them? How could that be?"

"That fire extinguisher was quick thinking on somebody's part," I said.

"Because they couldn't know for sure you'd go to the ladies' room?"

"Yes. Say somebody was waiting out in the hall, maybe planning to push me down the stairs. He or she sees me go into the bathroom. They run back here and get the fire extinguisher. Did you hear the door open?"

"No. But I was working in my office."

"Of course, the broom was right in the alcove. Still, it was quick and clever."

"And vicious."

"It was one of them. Tracy, or Fred, or Russell."

"I know. I'm not an idiot. But they've been with me a long time. Fred's been in this office six years. Russell's been here four years, and he was with me for two years before that when I was C of D North."

"I remember."

"And Tracy's been here three and a half years. They're all responsible, reliable people. You know, they're not the only staff people who've gone through this office. I've had maybe four or five others in the time I've been here who didn't work out for one reason or another. One enterprising gentleman was actually selling info to the media. I've watched these three and brought them along to where they could practically do my job."

"Not really."

He almost smiled. "Well, maybe not really. But I'd say any of the three could be moved into Bramble's job. They wouldn't do it quite as well, but they'd be better than anybody else I've ever had."

"I understand. But facts are facts."

"Oh, Lord."

"McCoo, there's something else."

"What now?"

"Tracy, Fred, or Russell—whoever it was—knew I wasn't leaving the building when I went to the bathroom. I didn't have my coat on."

"So?"

"So he or she knew that eventually you'd realize I'd been in the bathroom too long. You'd think I was sick or something and you'd come to check. You'd find the broom stuck through the door handle. You'd remove it and find my dead body."

"Yes—"

"Your fingerprints would be on the broom. You'd be the

first to find the body. You tell me, McCoo. What would you
think in a case like that?"

"Oh, my God!"

"Right."

"How can this get any worse?"

"I don't know."

"But it will. You realize," McCoo said, "that tomorrow at
nine the expanded round table convenes."

Then somebody knocked on the hall door, the door into the
outer office. I jumped. "They've come back to see if I'm
dead!" I said.

"Calm down. It could be anybody."

I stayed in McCoo's desk chair while he went through the
main office into the anteroom to the hall door. I heard him
mutter "Hummp?" as he saw who it was.

I heard the sound of the door opening. Then McCoo said,
"Paul," and I knew. It was Bannister. I stayed where I was.

"Harold." Bannister's voice was chilly.

"What's wrong?"

"I don't know that anything is wrong. But I'm going to
make sure it doesn't get worse."

"What are you talking about?"

"I thought it was only fair to tell you myself."

"Fair?" There was derision in McCoo's tone. He knew
something was coming.

"Yes, fair."

"Go ahead and tell me."

"I'm taking you off the bombing investigation, too."

Silence. After about thirty seconds, McCoo said, "Another
public relations move?"

"Not exactly. I want to be sure the investigation is done
right."

"Hey. What do I know? Twenty-five years on the job, and
part of it trained by you. I gotta be incompetent. Right?"

"That's not it."

"Go on."

"You know you've had a leak in your office?"

"Yeah. I'm a detective. I can figure out things like that."

"It's possible Officer Bramble was the leak."

"And?"

"And if she was, you might have wanted to stop her. Or you might have been furious with her."

"And?"

"You might have killed her."

· 25 ·

Quint, the FOP attorney who had been assigned to defend Daniello, said, "We stipulate that the officer is present voluntarily to aid the inquiry and does not, by answering any questions in this venue, relinquish any rights to later defend her actions in a court of law."

"We understand that, Mr. Quint," Deputy Superintendent Bannister said.

"And that this is an administrative proceeding; none of her testimony here later may be submitted to any civil or criminal court."

"Mr. Quint, you are aware of General Order 93-3 which states that the advice of counsel to decline to answer questions will not excuse an accused member from responding when he has been properly and lawfully ordered to do so by a member of higher rank."

"This officer has not been accused of anything. This is only an inquiry into the facts of the case. I would like to add that we have not received the Notification Re CR Investigation—"

"Which would be—"

"That would be CPD 44.217."

"Mr. Quint, this is a round table, not a criminal proceeding. The CPD wants to establish what happened to Officer Jurack. You're here to protect Miss—uh—Officer Daniello. Why don't we go ahead and see whether your client can answer the questions?"

"As long as we are aware that she does not abandon any of her rights as a citizen of this country."

I was pleased that Quint was doing the right things. The Fraternal Order of Police is supposed to defend cops in situations like this, of course, but back at the FOP ranch it would be grumbled about. Daniello had killed a cop; a lot of them would say that anybody who defended her was a turncoat.

I was less pleased with Bannister. His voice sounded properly regretful, but he looked puffed up and glossy with all the attention. Presiding at this round table might be his one final bid for the superintendency. Here he could be visible and commanding. I hoped he would be fair.

He rose, waiting until he had collected everybody's gaze. Bannister said, "On the record, now. I would like to introduce the members of this proceeding. I am Deputy Superintendent Paul Bannister. Also present, starting from my right, District Commander Kasmarczyk, Area Commander Ainslie, Assistant State's Attorney Sheets, Mr. Quint, Ms. Catherine Marsala, Mr. Lucas Vellie, Ms. Andrea Dawkins, and Mr. Philip Morganthaler."

The media as a whole hadn't been permitted in the room, but in the interests of appearing to the public to be hiding nothing, the department had decided to have Andrea Dawkins, who was a representative from the Battered Women's Coalition, Vellie, a representative from the mayor's office, and Morganthaler, a pool reporter chosen by lot. I had got in because Daniello was allowed two attorneys and one investigator. She had in fact one attorney and had chosen me as the investigator. I was listed as C. Marsala, and while Bannister recognized me when I came in, he hadn't said anything negative. I was with the FOP lawyer and Daniello, and besides that, I suspected Bannister in fact wanted as much press coverage as possible. Maybe he hoped I would write another piece about him—on how statesmanlike he had been during this difficult case.

Also, my very flattering portrait of him had appeared in this morning's paper. How could he lose?

The members of the round table were grim enough to have stepped out of a Daumier drawing. The commander of

Jurack's district, the Eighteenth, Al Kasmarczyk, sat gloomily behind the long table, head down, his bushy eyebrows shielding angry eyes. The head of Area Six, Commander Hamish Ainslie, was a grim Scot, with deep grooves running from his nose down to his chin, making him resemble a marionette. And the Assistant State's Attorney for the Felony Division, Marcus Butler, stared at the ceiling with his prominent, bloodshot eyes, unhappy to be involved at all.

The room was a perfect square, imperfectly painted cream over some drab green that showed through. Four very tall windows ran along one wall, like the windows in my old grade school. And they had the same pull-down tan fabric shades with cord tie-downs that my school had had too. This was not a glamorous building. Any time the city of Chicago wanted to cut loose funds for a new CPD headquarters was fine with me.

Outside it was raining. Cold rain. The perfect mood. The effects of the halon were long gone, but I felt subdued, as if there was a tragedy in the making.

Daniello sighed deeply.

"We're going to be somewhat informal here," Bannister said. "We'll call witnesses as they are available, and may ask Officer Shelly Daniello to respond more than once. I repeat: This is not a criminal proceeding."

Beside me, I heard Daniello whisper, "Right. It's worse."

"Officer Daniello, how long have you been a police officer?"

"Eleven years."

"And you went through the Chicago Police Academy?"

I could tell that Shelly wanted to say "Of course, you idiot" to Bannister, but she sat very still in the wooden witness chair and calmly said, "Yes, sir."

"And you had the usual training there, plus rookie training on the job after you graduated?"

"Yes, sir."

"Officer Daniello. In your training were you taught that an officer should wait to approach an offender until his or her partner is also in position?"

"Yes, sir."

"You did not follow this procedure in this case. Why was that?"

"My partner had exited our vehicle right behind me, and had followed me into the house. I didn't realize he had run into a perfectly visible wall."

"Did you look back to check?"

"No, sir, at that point I did not."

"And therefore he lost sight of you."

"I suppose he did."

"So he didn't know what situation he was getting into?"

"When I got to the television room, I called out 'Knife!' to warn him."

"Is that so? I'm not sure you mentioned that in the first round table. Now, Officer Daniello, are you aware of a training—uh, were you made aware during your training that an officer responding to a domestic or other situation with potential for violence must stop and listen? We call that the 'listen first' rule."

"Yes, sir."

"Did you do that?"

"I listened, but I heard Mrs. Jurack screaming in a way that I interpreted as being in extremis and in my judgment waiting would have put her life in jeopardy."

"Are you saying that of the stop-and-listen imperative, you listened but did not stop?"

"In the course of crossing the living room and kitchen, I had several seconds to listen to what was happening in the television room."

"Are you saying that of the stop-and-listen imperative, you listened but did not stop?"

"Yes, sir."

I thought, Bannister, you utter ass!

"And we are taught, are we not, that going into an unfamiliar situation, it is wise to pause and 'count four'?"

"Yes, sir."

"Did you ever think that your partner might be counting four?"

Mr. Quint, the FOP lawyer, said, "Now, I take it you knew this apartment well, Officer Daniello."

"Very well."

"And how many times would you say you'd been there?"

"Oh, a hundred? Two hundred. Too many to know for sure."

"And so you might say that it was not an 'unfamiliar situation'?"

"That's right."

"Officer Hubner, you've been partnered with Officer Daniello for some time?" Bannister said.

"Yes, sir."

"Now you must occasionally go to addresses that one or the other of you is familiar with? Bars you've responded to before? Places of business? Even homes?"

"Yes."

"Have you ever known Officer Daniello not to acquaint you with any information she had about the place you were going to?"

"No, sir."

"And did she this time?"

"No, sir. Not right away."

"How long was it from the time you got the call to the time she explained it was her sister's house?"

"We were at least halfway there."

*   *   *

"Officer Hubner," Quint said, "did Officer Daniello call out 'Knife!'?"

"Yes, sir, she did."

"You did not mention this before."

"I'm sorry, sir. I must have forgotten."

They went round and round. Although the FOP attorney was successful in getting reasons out of Daniello for what she did and doubts out of Hubner on some very minor matters, the big picture didn't much change. Daniello was in trouble.

"Officer Daniello, did you stop to think that by rushing into the room you call the television room, you placed yourself and ultimately your partner in a situation where you both could have been shot?" Bannister was smug.

"I believed it was necessary."

"Officer Jurack was a police officer and therefore known to own weapons and have experience in using them."

"But Ben Jurack had no history of using a gun against his wife," Daniello said.

"Did he have a history of using a knife against his wife?"

That stopped her. She had walked into that one. "No, this was the first time."

Too delighted to leave it alone, Bannister said, "Couldn't he have used a gun this time for the first time?"

"He could have. I didn't think he would. All you can do is go with what you know."

"Shouldn't you have waited until your partner arrived in the doorway with you, so as to present an overwhelming show of force?"

"In my estimation, with my knowledge of Ben Jurack's character, the presence of a male officer would have escalated the violence. Jurack despised women, and in front of a male officer he would have had to display even more dominance. Things would have only gotten worse."

"Things could hardly have gotten worse than they did, could they, Officer Daniello?"

Quint said, "I don't think that calls for a reply, Officer Daniello."

Daniello said, "He could have killed my sister and her child."

Quint said, "Officer Daniello, how much difference would it have made if you had stopped and listened and counted four and so on?"

"None. Ben Jurack was a police officer. This guy knew all the tricks too."

Bannister said, "We're going to take our mid-morning break now. Be back in this room in thirty minutes. We won't wait for anybody. After the break, I will call Dr. Emmy Suvitha."

We broke for late-morning coffee. Daniello and I went out into the hall. Hubner was standing talking with the pool reporter. When Daniello and Hubner locked eyes, neither said a word.

The lobby would be awash in reporters.

Daniello and I went down the back stairs, out a side door, through the alley, and across the street behind the CPD to a gyros place that had wonderful Greek pastries to go with the coffee. I ordered galatoboureko with mine. Daniello ordered baklava but cut her piece in two at the outset and gave half to me. She never tasted the half she kept for herself.

Behind her, a wall-mounted television was tuned to the local news, volume set low. But without hearing the words, I could read the block-printed headline:

CHIEF OF DETECTIVES REMOVED FROM BOMBING INVESTIGATION.

Daniello hadn't seen it, but I felt sick.

"I told you they'd get me," she said, stirring coffee.

"You handled yourself well."

"Did I make a real difference on the basic questions?"

"Um. No."

She sipped her coffee and put it down. She ate nothing.

A person who projected more sincerity than Dr. Emmy Suvitha would be hard to imagine. She considered each question gravely, pausing one or two seconds before responding. No one could possibly believe that she performed her autopsies sloppily, or left any part of them undone, or ever reached hasty conclusions.

"And after sectioning the bruised area, Dr. Suvitha, what did you do?"

"That gave me, you see, a type of cross-section that went down through the layers of skin and into the underlying muscle."

"And what is the purpose of this?" Bannister said.

"It is to see how deep the damage is."

"And was it severe?"

"I have prepared two enlarged color copies of the cross-section for your attention, one of the damaged area of the forehead, and one of an adjacent undamaged area. The structures are labeled. You will see the epidermis, or top portion of the skin. This is essentially tough and protective, and consists, from outside down, of the stratum corneum, literally horny layer; the stratum lucidum, the clear-looking part; the stratum granulosum; and the stratum mucosum. Under that is the dermis, or true skin. It contains connective tissue, but it is also rich in blood vessels, lymphatics, and nerves. You will also see running through it up to the surface sudoriferous ducts from the sweat glands and sebaceous ducts from the oil glands. The face is rich in sebaceous glands."

Quint said, "I am not certain that this testimony goes to who made that bruise."

Bannister said, "It will. Tell us about the damage, Dr. Suvitha."

"On the cross-section of the damaged area, you will notice

two types of leakage. The blood which has leaked from capillaries in the reticular, or deep, layer of the dermis. Also you will note patches of clear fluid, which is lymph. You will see also that in the section I am showing you, the sebaceous duct is damaged. It appears mashed."

"Dr. Suvitha," Quint said, "you call it mashed, which makes it sound like a lot of injury, but in fact this is a tiny structure, is it not?"

"It is. The entire bruise is one and one half inches long and less than a quarter of an inch wide. I have photographs."

"Let's let the doctor finish, Mr. Quint," Bannister said. He turned back to Suvitha. "Can you tell from this examination how long before death the blow was struck?"

"Deputy Superintendent Bannister! We don't know *any* blow was struck!" Quint said. "The man may have fallen and hit his head. One of the paramedics may have bumped him, in the course of loading him into the ambulance."

"This is not a courtroom. We're just trying to elicit information. Put it however you like. Dr. Suvitha, how long before death did the injury happen?"

"Perhaps more than a few seconds. You see these blood cells have begun to collect in little clots? And the pressure of the lymph and blood is distending the layers of the dermis. But the process is just beginning."

"More than a few seconds and less than . . . ?"

"Less than four or five minutes."

"And if I were to tell you that although the EMTs loaded him into their ambulance and took him to a trauma unit, they never were able to get a heartbeat, and the doctors in the trauma unit said he had probably been clinically dead when he was loaded into the ambulance, then would you guess whether this injury could have happened in the course of being loaded into transport?"

"It could not."

"And if I told you that Officer Daniello had been on the

scene for at least five minutes before Officer Jurack died, would you say, to the best of your medical knowledge, that this wound was made before she arrived on the scene?"

"It was probably not."

"Do you have any questions for Dr. Suvitha, Mr. Quint?"

"No, thank you, Deputy Superintendent Bannister."

"Officer Daniello. Did you notice a bruise on Officer Jurack's forehead as he came toward you?"

"No, sir."

"Officer Daniello, did you strike that man as he came toward you, stunning him, so that you could then execute him with a shot to the heart at point-blank range?"

"No, sir. I didn't."

Paul Bannister said formally, "It's now almost noon. I'm going to adjourn. Be back here promptly at one P.M."

I raced for the door.

I was in Marie Jurack's living room. Mr. Quint had taken Shelly to lunch, and I had made excuses.

"Do you know your sister is testifying before a court of inquiry today?" I asked Marie.

"Yes, she told me."

"Are you worried about her?"

"Of course."

But Marie Jurack had the same flat voice as before. She might care, but it certainly was hard to tell. I looked at one of the photographs on the lamp table.

"Who is that? Your husband?"

"Yes. That's Ben."

"And these are your parents?" An old walnut frame stood farther back, behind the lamp base, showing an aging photograph of an elderly couple.

"Yes."

"Ben looks a lot like your father."

"He does?"

"Yes. To me he does."

She didn't respond.

"Marie, Shelly tells me that your father was abusive."

"Well, he did have a heavy hand."

"Heavy hand? Does that mean he hit you?"

"He slapped us sometimes."

"And belittled you verbally?"

"Yes. He kind of did."

"So if Shelly came in while Ben was beating you or stabbing you, do you suppose she could have had a flashback to her father hitting her when she was a little girl? And might she fly into a rage and shoot him?"

Marie Jurack started to pleat a fold of her skirt, but her other hand grasped the fidgeting one and stopped it.

"No, I don't think so. She didn't do that."

"Experts say that abused women often put up with days of building tension and verbal abuse, then trigger the outbreak to get it over with. They say abusers are usually affectionate for a while afterward. I think when we talked you mentioned getting it over with."

She didn't answer.

"Was Ben affectionate after an outburst?"

"Sometimes. But not very."

"Did you trigger a fight to get it over with?"

"No. Didn't much need to. He always started it pretty well all by himself."

Good. She was showing a little spirit.

"And this 'fight' was worse than usual."

"That's true."

"And it was in front of Beanbag, too."

"That was wrong of him."

"Yes, it certainly was."

I looked at her and truly didn't know whether to feel sorry

for her or angry at her. She was so lumpy, so *unfinished* some-how in her droopy skirt, clunky shoes, cluttered baggy sweat-shirt.

But I knew what I had to do, and I had to do it now.

· 26 ·

Marie Jurack sat in the witness chair and stared at Quint and the hearing room with her eyes wide and her mouth partly open. Daniello stared, too.

"So you say you watched with horror, Mrs. Jurack," Quint said, "when Officer Daniello aimed her gun at your husband."

"Well, he was . . . I'm not sure. I don't like guns."

"Neither do I, Mrs. Jurack. But your husband had been a police officer for years. You'd seen his guns."

"Yes. He never let me touch them."

Had I done the right thing, bringing her? I've heard the expression for years that a person looked "like a deer caught in headlights." This was it, illustrated.

"At this point in time," Quint said, "your husband had just stabbed your arm to the bone. He had terrified your child. He had terrified you for years. You hated him."

"No. No, I loved him."

"You may have loved him. But it would be quite understandable if you also hated him. And now you were bleeding, and he cut your face and you knew you'd be scarred for life. And you loathed him—"

"No—"

"Officer Daniello shot him and he fell. Then she heard your daughter call out, 'Daddy!' She turned away to look at the child, horrified to realize that the little girl had seen her father shot. And he was down, lying on the floor, helpless at last."

"Please!"

"And you kicked him as hard as you could in the head."

*   *   *

I turned to Daniello with relief. Thank heaven Marie, however frightened, had been honest.

Daniello hissed at me, "You shouldn't have brought her."

"Shelly, she's helping you."

"She's hurting herself."

I could only see the back of Bannister's neck as he faced Marie, but it was rigid and arched backward. His shoulders hunched, like a man who wanted to punch something.

Marie was still in the witness chair. Bannister rose to question her.

I whispered to Daniello, "Maybe it's about time she took responsibility for her life. This is the first time she's really taken responsibility for events. In the long run, maybe she'll feel empowered."

"It's not worth hurting her."

"You have to fight these charges. You can't just cave in to them," I whispered.

"Look at her! She's totally humiliated!"

Marie clutched her purse to her chest. She still wore her shapeless sweatshirt, long skirt, and clunky shoes with heavy soles.

Shelly was right that she looked miserable.

"She'll feel better later," I said.

"Oh, sure! Do you realize she's going to be in all the newspapers? This is horrible!" Bannister looked angrily around at Daniello, who had spoken too loudly.

"That's not fair," I said softly. "She needed to do this."

"She'll be the woman who kicked a man when he was down."

"And high time, too, goddammit!"

"She'll feel like shit!"

"Just try to think how she would have felt after you were fired and maybe prosecuted criminally and she'd know forever afterward that she could have helped you and didn't."

"This is just one of the charges against me."

"One will help."

"Anyway, it's not me you're trying to help. It's your friend McCoo."

"You're my friend now, too. I hope."

"I don't think so."

Bannister put his fists on his hips. "Officer Daniello, I would think you could keep quiet, since it is on your behalf that we're holding this round table."

Daniello glowered.

Bannister said, "I have no questions for you, Mrs. Jurack."

When the break came, Daniello got up quickly, turned her back to me, and went to Marie. The pool reporter tried to talk with them, but Shelly grabbed Marie's arm and led her away fast, out of everybody's sight. Marie was crying. The pool reporter bolted to the phone in the lobby.

Deputy Superintendent Paul Bannister stalked out past me. His stiff gait and the cold glance he sent my way made it obvious that the brief goodwill I'd gained with the article was over. And it made something else obvious as well. He wanted to be superintendent so bad, it was like an aura around him. He hated it that McCoo had guessed right, even about this one point out of three.

"He doesn't seem to like you," Quint remarked. He gathered up his papers and his briefcase.

"Not anymore."

"Daniello seems mad at you, too."

"Sometimes you have to help people even if they won't help themselves," I said. I was sounding more like Sam every day.

Quint paused until I was looking him in the eye, and then said meaningfully, "Yes, you do." I liked him then, for wanting to make me feel better.

"How much does this help Shelly?" I asked.

"So-so. Not enough, I'm afraid."

"But at least she was telling the truth in this—"

"Ms. Marsala, she was still lying about the child being in the room and how close she was to Jurack when she shot him. Bannister's been making a big deal about her not telling Hubner right away that it was her sister's house and not pausing before she ran into the television room. But that's just stacking. Window-dressing. Plenty of police officers don't make the perfect decision in every instance. It's lying they really come down on like a ton of bricks. She might not know for sure how far away from Jurack she was when she fired, but if so, she should have said that. Personally, I think she does know, and they'll say she knew, that she misstated it in her first report and then was stuck with her lie. And the child, Belinda, was unquestionably in the room. That's a lie. They'll get her for that."

I didn't even try to go for coffee. I couldn't have swallowed anything.

"When did you first notice the child, Officer Daniello?"

"She must have just come into the room, sir. My sister was shocked and—and frantic. And right then I heard Belinda cry out or speak. And I turned and looked, and there she was in the corner, and she was walking toward Jur——um—her daddy."

"Officer Daniello. Can you now sit here and tell us that the child was really not in the room until then? You yourself were not far from the door. Where could she have come from?"

Daniello took a breath. Her shoulders squared, but her eyes were confused. "I just can't understand it, sir. But she wasn't there."

"Officer Hubner, you have testified that when you entered the room—which we are calling the television room—the child, Belinda, was already there?"

"Yes."

"And you testified you came in the only door?"

"Yes, sir."

"That was the door from the kitchen?"

"Yes, sir."

"I have a diagram of the apartment here, Officer. Will you indicate where you entered and where you stood?"

"Yes, sir."

"Let the transcript indicate that Officer Hubner showed that he passed through the kitchen, which has a back door and a door into the living room area, and he passed from there into the television room, which has only the one entrance. Is that right, sir, and did you see the child as you went through the kitchen?"

"She wasn't in the kitchen. She was in the television room when I got there."

"So it is your testimony that she was there all the time that Officer Daniello was there?"

"Unless she flew in the window."

"Officer Hubner, this is no time for jokes."

"I've been ballistics and firearms examiner for the Chicago Police Department for seventeen years," Lemuel Fox said.

Bannister asked, "And what are your qualifications? Where did you study?"

Quint rose impatiently, shaking his head. "Deputy Superintendent Bannister, we aren't in a court of law. Everybody here is willing to agree that the department firearms examiner can testify in department hearings. You're gilding the lily."

Bannister made fists of his hands but immediately relaxed. He said, "Good. Thank you. Mr. Fox, you tested the clothing of Officer Jurack?"

"I did."

"And what did you find?"

"I was given a white cotton undershirt to test. On it, in the front portion, was a small ring of powder and some metal flakes."

"A burned area?"

"Not really. Singed, you might say, but only very slightly."

"And what was your conclusion from this evidence?"

"That a firearm had been discharged near the shirt."

"How near?"

"Not closer than one inch and not farther than seven inches."

"And you're aware that various firearms and various types and even batches of ammunition result in various burn and powder patterns?"

"Of course, sir."

"How did you allow for that? How did you deal with that?"

"I was given a side arm labeled as being Officer Shelly Daniello's and containing the ammunition she allegedly used. I discharged the weapon at various standard distances to learn the performance of this particular weapon."

"And it is from that evidence that you formed your conclusions?"

"Yes, sir."

"Any questions, Mr. Quint?"

Trying to appear as if this were no more than he expected, Quint said, "No questions."

I studied Assistant State's Attorney Marcus Butler, Commander Hamish Ainslie, and District Commander Kasmarczyk. Butler's heavy lids blinked down over his bulgy eyes like a satiated toad's. He hadn't liked the whole case, but if it had to happen, he was glad it was so clear, so obvious. There would be no comebacks. Ainslie, unreadable, crossed his arms over his chest. Kasmarczyk, who had walked in angry, had relaxed, his bushy eyebrows now in a straight line, like resting caterpillars. He had come in afraid that Shelly Daniello would get away with it. Now, like all of us, he knew that, barring a miracle, she wouldn't.

*   *   *

In McCoo's outer office, there were sounds of drawers closing and chairs scraping. McCoo and I were drinking coffee—
Ethiopian sidamo, which McCoo said was less heavy than the
harrar and had a subtle lemon bouquet. A blue twilight was
deepening outside the windows. After I'd been there a couple
of minutes, Fred, Tracy, and Russell stuck their heads into
McCoo's office. "We'll say good night unless you need anything else?" Fred said. Fred was not his usual cheerful self.
Russell glowered at the world, and Tracy had frown lines that
she had not possessed a month ago.

McCoo looked at the clock. "I didn't realize it was past five.
Temperature's falling too," he said. "Bundle up. Wear layers."

Fred said, "Yes, den mother boss."

McCoo smiled wanly.

"Well, good night," Tracy said.

Russell said, "See you tomorrow, boss."

I waved, and McCoo said good night, but I know we both
felt extremely uncomfortable. "I really can't believe it's one of
them," he said. "I keep thinking there has to be some other
explanation. Somebody who lets himself in here at midnight,
something like that." A door slammed in the outer office.

"You said there were only two door keys, yours and Bramble's."

"That's right. But we're not Fort Knox. Security has one."

"McCoo, I really think you have to face facts. A stranger is
just terribly unlikely."

"Well, either way, I've fixed it."

"What?"

"I had the locks changed this morning. If anybody had a
key made, it won't work now."

"Hey, that's great!" I was delighted that he was fighting
back, even if he was locking the barn door after the horse had
been stolen.

Some more scraping, the coat closet slamming, and doors

closing. I heard McCoo sigh with relief. He wouldn't have to deal with Tracy, Russell, or Fred until tomorrow. It came home to me how much he must have suffered all day, working with three people and believing one of them had sabotaged him. And that one may have killed Bramble.

"Cat, how is the round table going?"

He'd been holding off asking. Fearing the worst, I suppose. I told him about Marie Jurack's testimony.

"That's great. How did you guess she kicked him?"

"Daniello kept describing her as dithering, hating Jurack, and at the same time saying Daniello shouldn't have shot him. If you had been beaten for years by somebody who was much bigger and stronger and was now lying helpless at your feet, what would you do?"

"If I felt a wave of hatred, maybe—"

"Plus the moment Jurack fell, Daniello realized Belinda was in the room. She looked away from Jurack to the child. She must have been frozen with horror for a few seconds when she saw Belinda was there. She wasn't looking at Marie."

"You know, that makes it all the more likely Daniello's telling the truth about not believing the child was there to begin with."

"You're right, it does. She was shocked to notice Belinda there."

"Will Bannister see it that way?" McCoo's voice went rough.

"Never. He scents victory. And sees himself as superintendent. Daniello said Belinda wasn't there. As far as Bannister is concerned, she lied."

"In that case, let's get to work."

"What do you have?" I asked.

"I've figured out the first reference to each leak in the Chicago newspapers. It took half the day. There must be a hundred different clippings here. The leaks get repeated over and over in all the papers, so I listed each reference by date and paper. Here are my sheets of notes. The circled date is the first mention."

"Okay." I pulled out my schedule of Bramble's work

assignments. "You've included the other two leaks, the fact that Jurack had a history of excessive force complaints on the job, and the fact that the department had commissioned that study of officers who beat their spouses."

"I figured I'd be thorough."

"Okay. But I'm not going to enter them on my chart because they were generally available in the office over a long period of time."

"All right."

He was holding himself together, but his manner worried me. Should I tell him his staff was worried, too, and why? How would it help to say they thought he was having memory lapses? It would be adding still another worry. I said, "Can you take a break or something?"

McCoo said, "I'm meeting Susanne for dinner. Going to the Bierstube."

"Oh, I'm glad."

"I'm not. I want to get this done once and for all. I'll be back right after dinner."

"You need some relaxation."

"I'll relax when we've solved this. But Susanne insisted on dinner. And when Susanne really insists . . ."

"I can imagine. Enjoy."

We walked out and we both glanced around the outer office. No one was there. I said, "McCoo, should we—um—shall we go through their desk drawers?"

"They deserve their privacy—oh, hell. I suppose we have to."

We did. McCoo looked like a man who had stepped in dog droppings, but we did it. Pens, pencils, coins, the FOP General Information Handbook, gum, candy bars, paper clips, discs, combs. Fred had extra photos of his kids and wife. Russell had a huge number of wrapped condoms, at which McCoo said, "Hmmm!" Tracy had a *Bride's* magazine. Fred had lottery tickets. Russell had a bottle of brush-on hair dye,

hidden under several copies of *Chicago Magazine*, as well as
Mennen Protein 21, Arrid, Hai Karate aftershave, Certs, and
Kiwi black shoe polish. Fred had Bufferin, Halls Vitamin C
Drops, Old Spice solid, Desenex, Propert's Leather and Sad-
dle Soap, Benadryl, Murine Ear Wax Removal System,
Pepto-Bismol, Phillips' Milk of Magnesia, and an envelope of
six twenty-dollar bills. Tracy had Pond's, Cellex-C skin care,
Noxzema, cinnamon-flavored dental floss, Cover Girl Instant
Cheekbones in sophisticated sable color, Max Factor Powder
Blush in mulled wine color, Vaseline Intensive Care, and a
Zagat's guide. They all had envelopes, paper, and a few
stamps. Tracy had a toothbrush and toothpaste.

"I quit," said McCoo. "There's nothing suspicious here."

"Right." I was disappointed; he was pleased.

"I'd better hurry. Susanne's waiting. I'm leaving you with one
key. If you go out for anything, lock the door behind you, so you
won't be attacked when you get back. Now look at this."

"This" was a shiny new deadbolt on the inside of the hall
door.

"I don't want any repetition of last night."

"Neither do I."

"When I leave," McCoo said, "bolt the door behind me.
It's a square bolt that can't be fudged with a credit card or
anything like that, so you'll be safe."

"All right. Good."

He went out. Through the glass in the door, he watched me
slide the bolt into place. Then he locked the door from outside with his key. He saluted me, and left.

I got a larger piece of paper from a yellow legal pad, so that I
could accommodate the extra information, sat at McCoo's
desk, and did my whole chart over again. Then I went through
McCoo's summaries and added the day of first publication of
each piece of leaked information:

	Staff	Leak appears in press:	Data reaches detective office from:
Sat March 8	Lupinski		First round table
			day after shooting
			(Hubner's statement)
Sun March 9	Shoemaker		
Mon March 10	Shoemaker, Koy	child present	
		at shooting	
Tue March 11	Lupinski, Koy, Shoemaker		autopsy report
			(bruise)
Wed March 12	Lupinski, Shoemaker		
Thu March 13	Lupinski, Shoemaker, Koy	bruise on	
		Jurack's head	
Fri March 14	Lupinski, Koy		CPD lab results
			(gunshot residue)
Sat March 15	Koy		
Sun March 16	Shoemaker		
Mon March 17	Lupinski, Shoemaker	shot near point-	
		blank range	
Tue March 18	Lupinski, Shoemaker, Koy		
Wed March 19	Lupinski, Shoemaker, Koy		
Thu March 20	Shoemaker, Koy		
Fri March 21	Lupinski, Shoemaker, Koy		
Sat March 22	Lupinski, Shoemaker, Koy		
Sun March 23	Lupinski, Shoemaker, Koy		

And then, of course, it was all perfectly, horribly obvious.

What now? Call McCoo at the Bierstube? No, let him have an hour of peace and relaxation. I'd wait for him to come back while I wrote up my conclusions, meanwhile worrying about how he would take this latest blow. I sighed. The office was so quiet, my sigh seemed to echo off the walls.

I rubbed my eyes with the heels of my hands, feeling very depressed. Who would have thought . . . ? But then, the answer would be hard to believe, whoever had done it. There was a slight sound. I raised my head.

And saw Tracy Shoemaker. She had a gun pointed at my chest.

· 27 ·

My heart missed a beat. Then it began to race.

"You can't shoot me," I said. "It would be as good as a confession. They'll trace the bullets to your gun."

"It's not my gun. I've been a cop for ten years, Marsala. I picked it up off a street guy a long time ago."

All right. So she would be willing to shoot me. But she'd probably rather not. Deserted as the building was, loud noises were never the best choice.

Tracy took a small cylinder from her pocket. Smugly watching me, she screwed it on the automatic.

Could I stall her long enough for McCoo to get back? Stall for a whole hour? Not very likely.

"Killing me won't help. They'll just figure out it was you the same way I figured it out."

"Oh, I don't think so. Bramble's hard disc was destroyed in the explosion. You've got the only original copies of the schedules. Hand them to me, please. Good. That's smart. I would have taken these sheets the day of the explosion, but damn Harold McCoo had to wait and go out last. Big hero."

"Bramble was your friend—"

"And then the next day, when we got back in here, the ATF and techies were in there all day, and then you and McCoo locked all that shit in the safe. Just think. If you hadn't been so fussy, you would have saved your own life."

"Bramble was your friend!"

"She wasn't friend enough to have covered for me."

"She wasn't dishonest enough to have covered for you."

"Stand up."

"You set a bomb to go off right near your own desk?"

"I thought that way nobody would suspect me. Anyhow, letter bombs are very selective. They're *so* selective I was afraid she might not be killed."

She poked me with the gun. I stood. I said, "They can reconstruct the schedule, just by asking everybody when they worked."

"Not really. We usually switched around some. And nobody is going to be able to prove where they were every day. Only Fred has a family. Russell lives alone. And Fred jogs and goes to the gym Sundays. They won't be able to get it exactly."

"The CPD paymaster will have a record. To cut your salary checks."

"Nope. He made it up from Bramble's disc when she sent it in to him. But the disc is history."

"Between McCoo and Fred and Russell—"

"You just don't get it. I don't think McCoo is even in shape to work it out. And a reconstruction is never perfect. Your list there's only a bunch of your ideas. Nobody can ever get me for this. Suspect me, maybe. Get me, no."

I believed utterly that McCoo would figure it out. She would not get away with it. But what good would that do me when I was dead? "You have the protection of a top cop," I said. "You won't need McCoo's support anymore."

"Damn right. Now walk ahead of me into the main office."

I did as she said. In the main office, the coat cupboard was ajar. She'd waited until Koy and Lupinski had left, and hidden in there. She saw me look at it, and smiled.

I couldn't run for the front door, unbolt the bolt, and unlock the lock before she shot me. Actually, I probably could not get two feet from the desk before she shot me.

"Okay," she said, "here's what I want you to do. Get up on that windowsill."

The sill was really a very wide shelf that ran along the window wall. Underneath it were the radiators. In the way of municipal things, the windows had not yet been replaced, and the sheets of plywood still covered the three windows that had been blown out. Slowly, as if my muscles ached, I climbed up on the sill. Actually, I was petrified both by fear and the fact that my brain was racing like mad. Not coming up with a solution, just racing.

"Now walk forward. That way."

I did, walking on the sill, until I was at the end of the line of windows. I was now in front of the window closest to the door, although it was not so very close, and between the main office door and the hall was the anteroom door. There was no way for me to run out and no point in even trying.

"Now you will notice that the plywood is in two pieces."

"Uh-huh."

The windows were so tall in this elderly building that one four-by-eight-foot sheet covered the top and another sheet, about three by four feet, covered the bottom.

"The bottom piece is loose," she said. "Just tacked on. Shoddy municipal workmanship."

"Uh-huh."

"If you leaned on it, you would fall out."

"Uh-huh."

"But first you will reach that top shelf of reference books just past my desk. You will pull a couple of them out and drop them on my desk. It's going to look as if you climbed on the ledge to get to the books on the top shelf, lost your balance, and fell out the window. Now we want your fingerprints on those books and the shelf, too, please—that's right. Pat the shelf. A little more. Good."

These offices were on the eighth floor. A fall of eight stories was surely fatal.

There was just one chance. Instead of waiting until she told me to jump, I shoved the plywood out the window. A gust of wet air caught the plywood and cold, wind-driven rain splattered me.

Desperately I tried to think what the outside of the CPD building looked like. The problem was I saw it almost every day, and therefore I didn't pay much attention to it.

I crept out onto the ledge outside, holding the window frame. Rain whipped my hair. I glanced back at Tracy, afraid she might push me.

"Hurry up!" she said. "Jump."

"Can't I have my last minute?"

I said this while trying to see the wall outside.

"No. Hurry up. I have to get out of here." She walked around the desk toward me.

I grabbed the window frame in my right hand and stepped out onto a narrow ledge. Icy rain drenched my neck.

The facade of the building was made of flat blocks, detailed at each floor with a horizontal ledge. The ledge was at most nine inches wide, a little less than the length of my shoes. It was just decoration. The blocks themselves were joined by mortar, the cracks between blocks two or three inches deep. A fingerhold at most.

I felt a sharp blow on my right hand, which still clung to the window frame. Tracy said, "Get going." Quickly, I let go and sidled as fast as I could to my left, along the ledge, facing the wall. I wished I were wearing shoes that were more solid, but I'd put on running shoes this morning.

Now I was out of her sight, and well beyond the last window of the detectives' office. I was clinging to the wall that formed the outside of the anteroom. Any second Tracy would realize she hadn't heard a scream and hadn't seen me fall.

Her head came out the window. I was four feet away, and in the rain it took her an instant to see me.

Her head ducked back in and a split second later reappeared with her hand and her gun. Keeping an eye on her, I crab-walked faster to my left. Then my left hand bumped into something.

My hand touched a downspout. It was metal and maybe ten inches in diameter. I hugged it and threw my left leg around it to its other side. Tracy fired, but the shot was high, hitting a block just over my head. Pieces stung my face.

I swung my body to the other side of the downspout. She couldn't see me now, but she knew where I was, and I thought the downspout metal wasn't thick enough to stop bullets from a .357. It might deflect them, though. I edged still farther away along the ledge.

A shot pinged off the downspout. Tracy swore.

For the first time I looked down.

Big mistake! On the eighth floor I was maybe eighty feet above the cement of the alley. The windows in some of the lower floors must have been lighted, though I couldn't see them directly, and there was a streetlight at the end of the alley that lit the pavement. The rain, as it fell past me, fell into light, and the trick of perspective made it look as if the lines of rain were converging, ending in wet shiny blackness that seemed a thousand feet below. I clung more tightly against the building, shaking.

Tracy climbed out on the ledge. She edged sideways and stepped over the downspout. My left side was away from her and my right side toward her. She was in the same position I was, facing the wall, which put her left side toward me, of course, and her right side away from me. She was right-handed and her gun was in her right hand, making it awkward for her to shoot me. Waytago! It was plain, dumb luck that things had arranged themselves this way. I hadn't planned it or even anticipated it.

Still, she had the gun. It was an encumbrance for climbing, but she only had to shoot me once.

She carefully held on to the crack between the blocks with her left hand and brought the gun hand across in front of her face, her elbow keeping to the right of her body, which meant that she couldn't get the gun farther than a position right under her chin. Not a good position to fire from, but all she needed was to hit me anyplace. I could hardly keep my grip as it was.

I scratched my hand around in the mortar crack. There was nothing there, but I bunched my hand as if I'd gotten hold of something, then quickly flung it sideways at her.

She flinched. It was just a tiny motion, but it caused her to sway back a little, away from the building. From sheer instinct, her right hand grabbed for the block, and she dropped the gun.

It landed between her chest and the wall.

Oh, hell!

Now her right hand let loose of the wall and inched slowly down toward her chest. She'd get the gun. No question.

I scrabbled as fast as I could toward her, got within two feet, careful to keep clutching with my fingers, and, making sure my left foot was as firmly planted as possible, I kicked her left leg.

She hadn't seen it coming; she had believed I was frightened into immobility. She gasped and grabbed for the wall. The heavy gun slithered down her chest, down her abdomen, between her legs, bounced on the ledge between her feet, somersaulted over the edge, and plunged away into darkness. I didn't wait to see. I was scuttling as fast as I could away from her. But I heard a distant dull thunk as the gun hit cement.

She was coming after me. She wasted no time grieving over the weapon. Every movement of her body was telegraphing: "Let's wrap this up."

We were now working our way sideways along the eighth-floor ledge. I was lighter and shorter than she was, which gave me a certain advantage under these circumstances. I didn't have quite as much weight to worry about and I could move a little more easily. On the other hand, she could move faster, and with a longer reach, if she ever got within arm's length or leg's length of me, she could hit me when I couldn't reach far enough to hit her.

And she was getting closer. A few feet to my left was the next downspout. I thought about shinnying down it, but realized just in time that would be a fatal mistake. She could get on it right after me and fireman-slide down on top of me and push me off with her feet.

My only chance was to go up. It was the only direction where my lighter weight would be any advantage.

I hugged the pipe. Because the building's blocks had large cracks between them, I was able to hold the pipe with my arms and push up with my feet, the running shoes helping somewhat because they had some give in them. It was almost like walking up a ladder, but much more difficult. It was awkward and after about ten "steps" my thigh muscles began to scream.

Tracy snarled when she saw what I was doing, but the instant she reached the pipe, she started to climb, too. I hoped the pipe was too weak to hold her greater weight and wished her section of it would loosen and crash to the ground, leaving my section attached. Oh, *sure*.

No such luck. Where was shoddy workmanship when you needed it?

Then again, if the entire thing came down, we would both fall to our deaths.

She tried to grab my ankle. I climbed higher.

I said, "How could you kill Bramble? You'd worked next to her for years."

The sound of her climbing, a scraping and grunting, came up to me but no words, until after half a minute she said, "I didn't want to."

There was a roughness in the answer that made me believe it. I kept climbing. It seemed to me the rain was growing less. I heard her say, "But she'd have told McCoo I was the leak."

"You murdered a friend."

"He promised me a promotion."

"Who promised you?"

She didn't answer.

"Winter?"

"Yeah, Winter. He promised me a promotion."

He seduced her.

"If I wasn't promoted now, I never would be."

I thought about what Louise Montoya had said, about how it was better in the department for women now, how they didn't realize or remember how bad it had been before, and yet how difficult it was still. I should have paid more attention.

"He promised you marriage," I said. She wouldn't answer.

Winter was divorced, the only one of the top cops who wasn't married. Another thing I should have paid more attention to.

I had reached the tenth floor, and could *not* climb any farther. My legs shook. My arms ached so much I was afraid I'd lose my grip on the pipe. There were windows about seven feet beyond the pipe. I let go of the pipe and started sideways on the tenth-floor ledge. Maybe I could break into one of the windows. Or maybe I could make it to the next downspout far enough ahead of Tracy to slide down.

As I worked sideways, my foot suddenly slipped. I panicked, clutched the cracks my fingers were holding, and slowly brought the foot back to the ledge. Feeling around with it, I realized there was a small patch of ice on the ledge. Ice? Where did that come from?

It gave me an idea.

I took my pen out of my jacket pocket. Usually I travel with as many pens and pencils as I can carry without embarrassing myself. It's from fear that I'll need to make important notes and not have anything to write with.

Tracy was now stepping from the pipe onto the ledge. Carefully, with my left hand, I leaned down and placed the pen on the ledge. I used my left hand because she wouldn't see what I was doing on the far side of my body, if she happened to glance over at me. But she was concentrating on not slipping.

I stepped cautiously over the pen, edged about two feet farther along, then put a pencil down. I stepped over that and inched still farther left.

There was another downspout ahead and beyond that were the two windows.

I slipped on another patch of ice. This time I was expecting it and had been making sure that one foot was firmly planted before moving the other. Only the front part of my foot would fit on the ledge unless I toed out. Pointed toward the wall, the front two-thirds of my foot would be on the ledge and the heel mostly off. It was awkward, hard to hold.

I cast a glance at Tracy. I watched her but kept my brain concentrating on my feet. Would she slip? My feelings were in conflict. I wanted to live, I wanted her to stop chasing me, but I had a kind of horror of seeing her fall, knowing I had killed her. As she inched toward the pen, I said, "Tracy, go back. Don't do this."

She didn't answer. Was I begging her because I really thought I could talk her out of it, or because I wanted to distract her, keep her from looking down at her feet?

"Tracy, please!"

She kept coming.

Then she slipped. It was just before she reached the pen. She slipped on the same patch of ice I had stepped on.

She went to one knee. Her fingers made claws on the edge of the blocks. Her other leg was bent awkwardly out to the side. She couldn't bend in the normal way; putting her knee in front of herself would push her off the wall.

She clung.

Then I saw her knee slip on the ice. The other leg couldn't hold her; it wasn't placed well. Slowly, very slowly, her fingertips slid on the blocks. Clutching wildly, she said, "Help me!"

Instinctively, I held my right arm out toward her. This was foolish, because I could not have reached her unless my arm were twice as long. And stupid because even if I had grabbed her hand, I could not have supported her weight. We would both have gone over.

Slowly the upper part of her body leaned backward. The tip of her right shoe was the last part of her to leave the wall.

And over she turned, shrieking as she fell through the dark and into the lighted air near the lower floors, and then with a thud, like dough on a breadboard, to the cement below.

My whole body shook. I trembled so hard that I hugged the pipe tightly, my face to the metal, to keep from being thrown off the ledge. For the first time, I realized how cold it was out here, and how cold I was. I was wearing indoor clothes, with Levi's, a thin knit shirt, and a blazer. I was chilled through.

I didn't look down again, but tried to assess my position. About five feet away from me was the first of the two windows. My left hand went to the crack above a building block. I took a grip on the block and it felt slippery. I looked at my fingers. The pads of the fingertips had been worn off by the rough blocks I had climbed. They were oozing blood. I might not be able to grip stone with them.

Then I felt the ledge with my foot. The sole of my shoe slipped.

The ledge was slick with ice. The two patches of ice had not been isolated incidents—and why should they be? The temperature was falling, and I realized with terror that while I had been correct that the rain had stopped, in fact it had changed to sleet. It didn't feel so wet because it was ice.

The entire building was glazing over.

The downspout pipe I held on to was becoming slick.

The ledge was glassy.

There was no way that I could reach that window, not even if it had been three feet away, instead of five. One step farther on that ledge, and I would slip to my death.

Forcing myself to think rationally, I realized that the only part of the ledge that was not glazed with ice was the part my feet stood on, the part that was protected by my feet. I would have to stay right here.

The pipe was icing over, and when I moved my shoulders, I could feel my jacket crack. There was ice on my shoulders. Ice was forming on my hair.

I would soon be too cold to hold on to anything.

I yelled "Help! Help! Help!" and then waited, listening for a response. I heard shouting. Looking around, I saw no one in the alley, and no window opened. Nobody looked out.

There was more shouting.

It was the lockup. The men's lockup was on the eleventh floor and the women's on the thirteenth. I had managed to climb to the tenth. Right above me, men were shouting and cursing in the cells.

Which meant nobody would pay attention to my calls, even if someone heard them.

Somebody would see the body in the alley and look up, wouldn't they? People ordinarily didn't look up, particularly if ice was falling in their eyes. But they would when they found Tracy.

But how soon would somebody happen to walk down the alley? It wasn't a thoroughfare and it wasn't the shortest route from the police parking lot into the building, either. It could be all night before anybody found the body.

Soon I would be too numb to hold on. Even if I didn't slip, how soon would I develop hypothermia and sink into unconsciousness? I'd better do whatever I could right now.

The downspout was not flush with the wall. Its brackets held it a few inches out from the stone. I wedged my left arm behind it. Then I pulled the shirtsleeve and blazer sleeve down over the arm all the way to the wrist, so that the skin of the arm was as insulated as possible. Up against cold metal pipe and with the circulation diminished because the arm was wedged tight, that part of my body was a prime candidate for frostbite. But if I lost consciousness, there was a chance I would still hang there, by the wedged arm.

McCoo would be back soon. He would see the plywood gone from the window, understand the situation, and find me.

But shouldn't he have been back by now?

Actually, shouldn't he have been back awhile already?

Oh, my God. McCoo had gone home. He'd had one of his

frequent memory lapses and just went home with Susanne after dinner. I knew he had. I knew he had.

My trembling grew worse. Soon I would stop trembling, and then I'd know I was sinking into hypothermia.

• 28 •

Time passed. After half an hour, I couldn't feel my left arm below the elbow. Both hands were numb. My feet were numb, and I had to hope that they were frozen to the ledge, because the muscles in my legs were trembling and not far from collapse. I started to envision myself found here in the morning, frozen and dead, hanging limp from the downspout by one wedged, bloodless arm.

Nobody came down the alley. Every once in a while I shouted, but nobody heard.

The sleet continued to fall. Someplace I had heard that sleet and freezing rain are not the same thing, but when I found myself really trying to figure out the difference, I realized that I had become semidelirious. I saw LJ and longed for him. I saw the interior of Jurack's house. It was almost as if I were there, except that firefly flashes hopped around in my peripheral vision. I was dying and hallucinating at the same time, watching Daniello burst into the television room, Jurack's knife flashing, Daniello raising her arm to fire, Jurack falling . . .

Then I thought, I know what happened at Jurack's. I know, and I'm going to die here and I'll never be able to tell.

My hair was a helmet of ice. My jacket was a hard sheath, and when I moved my right arm, ice cracked at the elbow.

And then I heard somebody say, "She's not here!"

Another voice said, "What's that down there?"

"Help!" I shouted, but they were yelling at each other. Two stories below and far to my right, somebody pointed out a window at Tracy's body, below me in the alley.

"Oh, God, no!" somebody said. It was McCoo.

"Help! I'm up here!" I screamed, but they didn't hear.

One hundred and fifty-seven years passed. Then I heard them down in the alley. Somebody said, "It's Tracy Shoe-maker!"

"Up here!" I screamed at the top of my lungs. I screamed so loud my voice cracked and when I tried to scream again, I couldn't make a sound.

But they'd heard me.

"What happened?" I asked McCoo.

I was sitting in Fred Koy's chair in McCoo's main office. I couldn't stop shivering, and part of my left arm was beginning to feel as if it had been scalded.

Susanne McCoo stood next to him, looking like a woman who had dressed hastily, her hair ruffled and part of her blouse coming untucked from her skirt.

A uniformed officer said, "The boss got here a few minutes ago, looking like he'd been drug through a hedge backward."

"I'll tell you what happened," Susanne said.

At 11 P.M., according to Susanne McCoo, Harold McCoo had sat bolt upright in bed and yelled, "Oh, my *God!*" frightening her, she said, out of a year's growth. She added with a soft laugh, and a gesture at her rounded body, "If he could frighten me out of five years' growth, I'd be even better off."

The paramedic, who was wrapping a Mylar space-age thin silver blanket around me, told McCoo that my "core temperature" was low and they were going to take me to the hospital. I said no. He said yes. I said no. Susanne said, "Set my husband a good example," and I decided okay.

"I'll go but I need to do one thing first."

I dialed Hal Briskman at the paper. For the first time in my memory, he wasn't there. Sure, it was nearly midnight, but I'd called him later than that a lot of times. Maybe he was getting old. I'd have to remember to charge him with that when I felt better. Right now I was feeling as if beetles were gnawing at my muscles and my organs.

I called him at home.

"Hal?" I said.

"Cat? I hope this is important."

"It's important. Hold the Winter interview. He's guilty."

I told them what Tracy had said about Winter. As they trundled me out the door, I remembered my ideas and grabbed McCoo's sleeve.

"I think I've figured it out."

"What out?"

"What happened at Ben Jurack's house."

"Tell me."

"Listen, it was the window when bobble did Beanbug in was in because the gun wouldn't unless—"

"What's happening to her?" McCoo yelled.

I tried to explain. "The body is only evilly con-confused isn't dead but Shelly fired bobble when the ice happened ice nice shoot shoot loot—"

"We call this hypothermia," the EMT said.

Eight forty-five in the morning at the Chicago Police Department. I felt fifty years younger than last night, when I'd felt a hundred and fifty years old.

The first person I saw in the corridor outside the round table hearing room—other than a gauntlet of reporters who were begging me to talk with them—was McCoo.

"I've been waiting for you," he said. "Are you okay?"

"Actually, I'm not bad at all. Not once I got warm and got fed some hot soup and then got some sleep. There's a prob-

lem here—" I showed him the inside of my left forearm from
elbow to wrist. It had turned a blotchy red-purplish color.
"They think it's frostbite."

"What are you supposed to do about it?"

"Wait a few days and see. Keep it dry. Let it have air. If it's
frostbite, they say it may form a 'black carapace,' which
sounds like I'm turning into a cockroach, but it's supposed to
be a good thing. That could last several weeks, but when it
falls off, there may be perfectly good skin under it. My happy
consultant told me there's an old frostbite saying: 'Freeze in
January; operate in July.' So even if it needs a skin graft, we
won't know until a lot later."

"Let's get out of this mob. I can hardly hear what you're
saying."

We made it into a narrow, windowless corridor that ran
behind the courts, a passageway that the judges use. It was off
limits to the press. There was an alcove with a water fountain.
We huddled there.

McCoo said, "You're in all the papers."

"I know. I was a celebrity at the hospital. Every nurse and
orderly and doctor thought they were the first one to realize
why I was there."

"Haven't you seen the articles?"

"Couldn't stand to look at them."

"*Chicago Today* is particularly gleeful."

"I'm not surprised. Do they link me with you?"

"Not explicitly. They say you were in my office investigating the source of the leaks. But they're so focused on Tracy
and the bomb, why you were there kind of gets overlooked.
'Cop Plants Bomb' is the big headline. 'Deputy Superintendent Winter Involved in Bombing' is very big too."

"What's happened to our Gregory Dennison Winter?"

"He's under arrest. He claims he never asked Tracy to blow
up Bramble. He won't admit he was even the leak. They found
an undeposited check from him at Tracy's home. A lot more

evidence is coming out. Bank deposits. Notes. Her mother, a Mrs. Leggitt Shoemaker, is saying Tracy left an envelope for her to hold."

"Fine. McCoo, look at me. You're saying this all very upbeat, but in fact it doesn't help you much, does it?"

"Oh, I don't know . . ."

"Yes, you do. So Winter was the maggot in the apple. They'll still say you had a leak in your own office and never knew it."

"That's exactly what I did have."

"Unfair as it is, it looks like you were lax."

He stopped his cheery talk and his gaze went inward. McCoo was too honest a man to give an easy answer. "I am personally very relieved," he said slowly. "I know what happened now and who did it."

"Yes, but your reputation is no better off. And, far worse than the leak, there's still Daniello shooting Jurack."

"Right. Cat—last night, before you wigged out, you started to say you'd figured out what happened."

"I remember."

"You remember saying it or do you remember your solution?"

"I remember my solution."

"Then I'm going into the meeting with you."

"You aren't one of the permitted audience."

"Tough. I'm gonna be there."

"But I thought we weren't going to let them know you knew me."

"I'm not only gonna be there, I'm going in to make sure they listen to you."

"But I haven't told you my idea yet."

"I don't care. I have faith in you. Plus, you've been standing up for me long enough. Now it's my turn."

"You'd risk your reputation? Without even hearing what—"

"Piece of cake."

*   *   *

"I guess the Chicago Police Department owes you a vote of thanks, Ms. Marsala," Bannister said, while he adjusted his papers on the table in the hearing room. I wondered why he looked so relaxed and pleased, when McCoo had not yet been removed as a rival. Then I realized that at least Winter had been removed, permanently, and that cut Bannister's rivals down from four to three. Now all he had to do was destroy McCoo, and Bannister would be looking good for the top job.

McCoo said, "Ms. Marsala has something to say to the round table."

"Oh, I'm afraid we can't permit that, Chief McCoo. She's not a witness to anything."

"She has something to say that you need to hear."

The rest of the round table participants were edging their way inside. The two other top cops, Area Commander Hamish Ainslie and District Commander Kasmarczyk, walked army-straight, heads up, but their eyes were troubled. The morning's news had hit them hard.

Assistant State's Attorney Marcus Butler's heavy-lidded eyes were half closed. He had just run the press gauntlet and his face was still set in a "no-comment" freeze.

The press pool rep and the other observer followed. Both were rumpled and unhappy. Finally, Shelly Daniello and the FOP attorney, Quint, entered. Shelly caught my eye for just a second. Then she gave me a minute nod. Quint pushed the door tightly closed. The noise from the hall faded.

"Ms. Marsala has something to say," McCoo repeated.

The atmosphere in the hearing room twanged with sudden tension. Quint froze in his tracks. McCoo and Bannister faced each other, both tall men, both so deeply angry that their faces showed no expression at all.

"You're out of place, McCoo," Bannister said. "And out of line. You don't belong at the round table." Bannister was McCoo's direct superior. He could command McCoo to shut up and McCoo would risk dismissal by refusing. Bannister was seconds from barking such an order. Ainslie, Butler, Daniello, and the others stopped cold where they stood.

McCoo said, "You and the department owe this woman—"

"I'm certain we owe her a great deal. This is not the place to pay that debt."

"—owe her attention. But more important to you is that she can go to the press with what she has deduced. If you've made some uninformed decision in the meanwhile, you're gonna look like an id——"

Surely McCoo was about to say Bannister would look like an idiot. He caught himself with almost visible control, and said, "—like you had made a hasty decision."

Bannister thought fast. We waited. Maybe I'd misled McCoo, maybe my explanation would fall on its face, and it seemed so simple—

So simple there had to be something wrong with it?

"McCoo, you'd better be right, or you're in deep trouble," Bannister said, quietly enough that only McCoo and I could hear.

He turned to the others. "Would you excuse us for about ten minutes? We need a short conference."

"Not just us," McCoo said. "Quint and Daniello, and Ainslie, Butler, and Kasmarczyk."

"And Brad Hubner," I said.

Somebody fetched Hubner from an adjacent room where the witnesses waited.

Ainslie was stony. Kasmarczyk was furious. If the light in the room had echoed the mood, it would have been blood-red. When they were seated, Bannister said in a voice all of a single pitch, "Get on with it, Ms. Marsala."

I glanced at McCoo. He smiled at me, probably hoping to encourage me. I swallowed.

"Um, Officer Hubner."

"I can't hear you, Ms. Marsala," Kasmarczyk said, making no effort to control the nasty edge to his voice. "Please stand up."

McCoo said, "You can't—"

But I quickly said, "Fine." I wasn't a police officer, so he couldn't order me around, but it wouldn't help for McCoo to tell Kasmarczyk so.

I said, "I'm going to discuss the question of the child, Belinda, being in the room when Officer Daniello fired the shot that killed Jurack."

"Shot that killed *Officer* Jurack," Bannister said.

"If you wish. Now, Officers Daniello and Hubner, listen and tell me if I'm wrong. School was just out; you've said over and over it was a bright, cheerful day. When you ran into the house, Officer Hubner, you were wearing dark glasses, and you crashed into a wall."

"That's right."

"But as soon as you took the glasses off, you could see perfectly well."

"Yes, of course."

"Officer Daniello. You had *not* been wearing dark glasses. When you ran into the house, you were going into a house you knew well?"

"Of course." There was a glimmer of light in her eyes as well as she answered.

"So you ran through rooms you knew, into the television room, which was even darker. We've all been told the shades were partly pulled."

"Yes."

"Your familiarity with the house kept you from realizing that you had come from a bright, sunny day outdoors into a dim house and into a darker room. A room with the shades half drawn."

"Of course!"

"You talked about light 'glinting off the blade' of the knife Jurack held. You would not have said that if the whole room had been brightly lighted and you could see it well. When you fired at Jurack, you had not seen Belinda in the corner because you *could not* see Belinda. Your eyes hadn't adjusted to the dark. When Hubner came in, he saw her immediately. And after the shooting, when you heard her speak, it was a minute or two later. You turned, saw her, and assumed she had just entered, because as far as your eyes were concerned, you were seeing her for the first time."

Daniello gripped the edge of the table.

"By then your eyes had adjusted."

I didn't look at Bannister. I could feel the anger radiating from him and Kasmarczyk, but I stared only at Daniello's white knuckles. There was half a minute of silence, and then Quint said, "Well, hey!"

"Of course we still have her lie about her distance from Jurack—" Bannister said, and then stopped, realizing he was giving himself away.

I said, "No."

There was silence.

"Officer Daniello," I said. "Am I right in thinking you don't have a handgun now?"

"That's right. They took it for tests."

I was going to ask for McCoo's, but then my anger at Bannister got the best of me, and I thought, Stick it to the bastard.

"Deputy Superintendent Bannister, if you were to unload your side arm, could we use it to demonstrate something?"

He couldn't say no. It would have looked churlish.

Very sullenly, he took out an automatic. There was no round in the chamber; he checked. Then he removed the magazine, and instead of unloading the magazine, reassembling it, and handing me the empty gun, he dry-fired the thing once, as if to be especially thorough, and then handed it to me with no magazine in it. It felt too light, but that probably wouldn't make any difference.

I said, "Officer Daniello, would you stand up, please?"

She did and I handed her the gun.

"I am Ben Jurack," I said. "I'm going to ask you to turn around, away from me. Then turn back when I tell you to. That will simulate your coming into the room."

"Okay."

I walked to a place about ten feet from her. "Did you have your gun out as you came into the room?"

"No. I brought it out when I saw the knife."

"All right. Do exactly as you did then. Now turn away from me." She tucked the gun in her waistband. I picked up a pencil to be the knife.

"Now turn back."

"Freeze!" she said.

"Oh, it's the sister!" I said, stalking a step toward her.

"Knife!" she said. "Drop that knife!"

I went one more step. I was about six feet from her and I raised the "knife" and stepped one half step closer. She was deep in reliving the moment, and anger tightened her face. "Drop it!" she yelled, and as I lunged, she brought up the gun, arms extended in perfect Weaver position, and fired.

It clicked. "Hold that pose!" I said.

She was just under four feet from me. Her arms were extended fully out. She was tallish; her arms were roughly two and a half feet long. The gun extended six inches.

"Now where's the gun muzzle, Deputy Superintendent Bannister?" I asked.

Daniello said, "Oh, my God!"

"This is scandalous!" McCoo shouted from my kitchen.

Susanne McCoo and I exchanged glances. Neither she nor McCoo had ever visited my place before and he had decided to make coffee for the three of us while we waited for the pizza to be delivered. We should just sit down and rest, he said. He'd do all the work. It turned out I had the wrong kind of pot, and my coffee was pre-ground.

"Never let anyone grind your coffee for you," he shouted.

"Pretend you're in the Gulag," I said. I didn't have to shout, nor did he. My kitchen opens directly out of my living room and McCoo wasn't more than four feet from the back of the sofa.

"Where's the spring water?" he yelled.

I said to Susanne, "It must be so nice to have him back to his old self again."

"It's heaven," she said, only half-ironically, putting her feet up on my ottoman, which did not match my sofa, which did not match my chair, which did not match the draperies.

"Where's the spring—"

"I don't own any!" I yelled back.

"Do you mean I have to use *tap water?*"

"Yes."

Silence for a few seconds. Long John Silver flew down and sat on my shoulder. I had told the McCoos his history and how good a talker he was. After which he had not said one word. Finally there was McCoo's voice from the kitchen.

"Where's the cream?"

"Don't have any."

"Where's the half-and-half?"

"Don't have any. Use milk."

"Have you no pride?"

I didn't dignify that with a reply.

Dead silence from the kitchen. The ominous quiet lasted about five minutes. Susanne McCoo and I used the time to relax.

"It was so obvious," McCoo said. "Of *course* a well-trained careful officer like Daniello would use the position she'd been trained for when she shot. How could I have been so blind?"

"People don't think of everything. The Maya had wheels on their children's toys and never thought of using them for work carts."

"It was so obvious."

"Plus, you weren't thinking that way. You're used to using ballistics to figure out who fired the gun from where, or was the gun close enough to the victim for a suicide."

"No. It was obvious. I should have seen it."

"Actually, it was all my fault," I said. "We had all the information we needed days ago. I should have thought of the staffing chart immediately. Bramble hinted at it when she and I had lunch together."

"Well, why didn't you?" McCoo said.

"Harold!" Susanne said. "It's *not* Cat's fault. Or your fault. Why do you have to be so rude?"

"Cat's used to me."

"I'm used to him."

"Anyway," McCoo said, "I'm not rude. I'm just outspoken."

"Like that's different," Susanne said.

The pizza arrived. I went downstairs and got it. By the time I got back to the third floor, Susanne had three plates out.

*　　　*　　　*

"I'm going to write an exclusive on this for Hal," I said, trying unsuccessfully to keep a long string of cheese from landing on my nose.

"Good," McCoo said.

"And he's going to pay me serious money."

"Good."

"You know my reporter friend Barney Ellerway? Who do you think is his Deep Throat in the department?"

"We'll probably never know. But I'd guess Louise Montoya."

"Really?"

"Yes. She thinks the department should be more open to the public, anyhow. And it hasn't been easy working under Spurlark."

Long John still wasn't talking. "Say 'To be or not to be,' LJ," I begged him. "Impress the guests."

The cheese landed on my wrist.

"Why kill Bramble?" McCoo asked.

"The first day I came to the office, as I was leaving, Bramble sent Russell and Fred on an errand to pick up papers at one of the districts. Why both of them? Wouldn't one be enough? That left her and Tracy in the office. Then she left and walked all the way to the *Chicago Today* building to deliver me the photocopies. That left Tracy alone in the office. Bramble had noticed that the leaks in the newspapers, the three major leaks, had come out the day after Tracy had either been in the office alone, or with just one other staffer. When it's you and another person, you get time alone to go into files that aren't your business, because sooner or later that other person will go to the bathroom or go to lunch."

"I was there," McCoo said.

"Sure, but in your own separate office."

"True."

"Look at the chart. Hubner testifies at the first round table that Belinda was there when Jurack was shot. It gets to your office on March 8, and it is in the papers by March 10. Tracy was staffing your office alone on Sunday, March 9. The autopsy results, the ones that contain the results on Jurack's head wound, hit your office on March 11. Fred, Tracy, and Russell are all in the office. No leak. The next day, March 12, it's only Tracy and Russell, and on March 13 the first leak about the head wound comes out. On March 14, the results come in from the lab about the distance from the gun to Jurack. Fred works Saturday the fifteenth. Nothing in the press on Sunday. Tracy works Sunday the sixteenth. Monday, March 17, the leak is in the papers."

"Yes. Well, we know *now.*"

"Tracy didn't want to make it obvious, by taking stuff only when she was alone there, but she was under pressure. She was between a rock and a hard place. Winter needed the leaks to keep coming, to keep up interest in the case."

"It really wasn't obvious at all," he said with some heat. "I didn't notice."

"Well, I think Bramble wasn't sure either. And she didn't want to be unfair. So she decided to plant that false sheet about Daniello's blood alcohol and see if Tracy bit. She got rid of Fred and Russell, put the sheet on her desk, and left to meet me. But what she actually accomplished was the opposite of what she wanted. It told Tracy that Bramble was on to her. So she sent Bramble the letter bomb."

"So why didn't Bramble tell me?"

"Well, I imagine—um—frankly—oh, hell, cancel the 'frankly' part."

"Because I was acting like such a baby. Is that what you want to say?"

"Not exactly. You'd had a series of blows. You were being sabotaged repeatedly by one of your friends. Somebody you knew and liked and had reason to think valued your friendship. Bramble didn't want to add to that. She wanted to find out for sure first. You'd chosen Tracy for the job. It was a respected position. She should have been grateful to you."

"Gratitude doesn't work. When somebody is beholden to you, they're likely to resent you."

"True. Nevertheless, Tracy owed you. It's friendly in your office. Bramble knew this was going to hurt you."

"She couldn't let the leak go on."

"No. Of course not. She would have told you when she knew for certain. She underestimated Tracy."

"That poor, poor child," Susanne said.

"Bramble was very devoted," I said.

"I meant Tracy," Susanne said. "Her life must have been empty."

McCoo said, "But if the press had got hold of the blood-alcohol thing and leaked it, it would have made Shelly Daniello look really bad."

"For a day or so. Once Tracy leaked it, Bramble would have found some way to tell the media it was bogus, for all the reasons you told me. Dr. Suvitha would certainly say she had never drawn any of Daniello's blood. It wasn't her signature on the sheet. The Medical Examiner's Office would say that they never analyzed any blood but cadaver blood. Especially not from a police officer. Daniello would confirm that she had not been asked to give blood. Even Cleary and Bannister would have to admit that procedure did not allow the ME's Office to draw blood from live suspects. The report would be totally discredited. Come to think of it, the only person who'd get stuck was the reporter. The competing papers and TV would pounce on the mistake with glee. It would go a good way to discredit all the earlier leaks, too."

"Maybe. Maybe some mud would cling to Shelly Daniello's reputation."

"I'm afraid Bramble was willing to risk Daniello's reputation for yours, McCoo."

"Lord."

"Next, Bramble would tell the department that she had left the paper on her desk as a test trap and that Tracy had fallen into it."

"That could get Bramble in trouble."

"How much trouble? She didn't publish it. She didn't promulgate it. She didn't even put it in Daniello's file. She left it in what should have been a secure place, the desk of the secretary to the chief of detectives. The persons who promulgated it were Tracy Shoemaker *and a deputy superintendent of the Chicago Police Department.* By implication, they'd better find out which deputy superintendent it was."

"I still say she could get in trouble."

"I still say it would look extremely unfair if she were punished when a top cop was the bad guy."

"Nevertheless, they might have punished her."

"She was willing to risk that for you, too, McCoo."

"Want to see the evening news?"

McCoo said, "Yeah! This is the first day in two weeks I could watch and not wince."

We turned on Channel Two. We saw the handsome face of Larry Spector. Long John flew over and sat on the TV.

"—this finally the end of winter?" Larry asked Channel Two's weatherman Dave Forrester.

"Well, Larry, it may be. We have a high-pressure cell building in from the west. There will be a wind of twenty to thirty miles an hour tomorrow, but the cold, wet weather is gone for now. More later in the newscast."

Long John finally uttered. He said, "Poor, poor dumb mouths!"

Susanne smiled delightedly. McCoo said, "Pass the thin crust."

I did.

"And the hot pepper, too," he said.

"Chicago police announced the closing of their inquiry into the shooting of Police Officer Ben Jurack. Deputy Superintendent Paul Bannister made the announcement in a news conference at Eleventh and State—"

There was a set-up view of Bannister in the first-floor hall of the CPD building. He stood in front of the wall of stars belonging to officers killed on the job. Go for it, Paul.

"We are extremely pleased to find that Officer Shelly Daniello acted responsibly in her confrontation with Officer Jurack," he said, looking like a man who had swallowed a sea urchin.

"Does this mean Chief McCoo is off the hook?" a reporter yelled.

"We are equally pleased that Chief McCoo saw his way so quickly to the—what happened—um—certainly one of our most experienced and astute administrators," said Bannister, clearly wishing the sea urchin had been cyanide. ". . . credit to the department," he finished up.

"Hooooo," said Susanne McCoo.

"Lardbrain," McCoo said mildly.

McCoo had forgiven Bannister, claiming that he was under a lot of pressure. I hadn't forgiven him, and didn't plan to.

With an inset of the bomb damage to his right, Larry Spector said, "Also at the Chicago Police Department today, Superintendent Spurlark confirmed that Deputy Superintendent Gregory Dennison Winter has been relieved of his duties as a result of his involvement in the bombing of—"

Now we saw a shot from a high angle of Spurlark and Bannister, the angle making them look small, two heads surrounded by the heads of a pod of reporters.

Finally, there was a shot of a car approaching the Criminal Courts Building. Reporters ran to catch up. Uniformed officers held them back while two Cook County sheriff's deputies got the prisoner out of the car. Debby Leeds, Channel Two co-anchor, provided a somber voice-over, explaining the arraignment procedures. But of course none of us needed the voice-over to know who this was.

It was the man who had sabotaged McCoo while pretending to be his friend. The man who had dangled irresistible bait in front of a troubled, selfish young woman. The man who had set in train the events that would murder Bramble.

Even as he was led inside to meet an ugly, well-deserved future, Gregory Dennison Winter looked so good. Chiseled, aristocratic features. Upright stance. And still wearing his well-cut, high-priced, light wool suit—two suits like that would cost as much as a car. The outside of Gregory Dennison Winter looked wonderful.

I thought: You were right, Bramble. You can wrap a fig in foil, but that doesn't make it chocolate.

ABOUT THE AUTHOR

In addition to her Cat Marsala series, Barbara D'Amato is the author of the Anthony and Agatha–winning true crime book *The Doctor, the Murder, the Mystery: The True Story of the Dr. John Branion Murder Case*, as well as a mystery novel, *On My Honor*, which was nominated for an Anthony in 1990. Her musical comedies have been produced in London and Chicago. She is a past president of Sisters in Crime International and also of the Midwest Chapter of Mystery Writers of America. She lives in Chicago, Illinois, and Holland, Michigan.